Therapeutic Problems
in Pregnancy

Therapeutic Problems in Pregnancy

EDITED BY

P. J. Lewis
Clinical Pharmacology Unit,
Institute of Obstetrics and Gynaecology,
Queen Charlotte's Hospital for Women,
London

University Park Press
Baltimore

Published in USA and Canada by
University Park Press.
Chamber of Commerce Building.
Baltimore. Maryland 21202

Published in UK by
MTP Press Limited
St Leonard's House.
Lancaster. Lancs.

Library of Congress Cataloging in Publication Data
Therapeutic problems in pregnancy.

    1. Pregnancy. Complications of. 2. Pregnancy.
Complications of - Chemotherapy. 3. Fetus. Effect of
drugs on the. I. Lewis. P. J.
RG572.T45   618.3'061   77-6317
ISBN 978-94-011-7929-4   ISBN 978-94-011-7927-0 (eBook)
DOI 10.1007/978-94-011-7927-0

Contents

List of Contributors   vii

Foreword: *C. J. Dewhurst*   ix

PART 1: HYPERTENSION IN PREGNANCY

1 The use of antihypertensive drugs in pregnancy: *L. J. Beilin and C. W. G. Redman*   1

2 Antihypertensive drugs and uterine blood flow: *D. F. Hawkins*   19

3 The effect of antihypertensive drugs on the fetus: *G. S. Dawes*   35

4 Fetal outcome in pregnancies complicated by severe hypertension treated with propranolol: *G. M. Stirrat and B. A. Lieberman*   45

5 The management of hypertension in the pregnant woman: *P. J. Lewis, M. de Swiet, G. V. P. Chamberlain and C. J. Bulpitt*   53

PART 2: CARDIOVASCULAR THERAPY

6 Heart disease, parturition and antibiotic prophylaxis: *Rosalinde Hurley*   69

7 Drug treatment and prophylaxis of thromboembolism in pregnancy: *M. de Swiet, Elizabeth Letsky and Heather J. Mellows*   81

PART 3: MEDICAL DISORDERS

8 Thyroid therapy in pregnancy: *I. D. Ramsay*   93

9   The drug treatment of epilepsy in pregnancy: *A. Hopkins*   103

10 Epilepsy, anticonvulsants and abnormal babies: *S. R. Meadow*   109

11 Diabetic therapy and pregnancy: *Nina Essex*   117

PART 4: DRUGS AND THE FETUS

12 Maternal drug therapy and enzyme induction in the fetus and
    newborn: *D. S. Davies and A. R. Boobis*   127

13 Maternal drug therapy and neonatal jaundice: *Louise A. Friedman
    and P. J. Lewis*   141

14 The influence of maternal drug administration on human fetal
    breathing movements *in utero*: *K. Boddy*   153

    Index   163

List of Contributors

L. J. BEILIN, MD, FRCP
Reader in Clinical Medicine,
Department of the Regius Professor
  Medicine,
Radcliffe Infirmary,
Oxford

K. BODDY, MB, MRCOG
Senior Lecturer in Obstetrics and
  Gynaecology,
University of Edinburgh

A. R. BOOBIS, BSc, PhD
MRC Research Fellow,
Clinical Pharmacology Department,
Royal Postgraduate Medical School,
London

C. J. BULPITT, MSc, MD, MRCP
Senior Lecturer in Epidemology,
London School of Hygiene and Tropical
  Medicine,
London

**G. V. P. CHAMBERLAIN, MD, FRCS,
  FRCOG**
Consulting Obstetric Surgeon,
Queen Charlotte's Hospital for Women,
London

D. S. DAVIES, BSc, PhD
Reader in Biochemical Pharmacology,
Clinical Pharmacology Department,
Royal Postgraduate Medical School,
London

G. S. DAWES, DM, FRS
Director,
Nuffield Institute for Medical Research,
University of Oxford

C. J. DEWHURST, FRCS Ed, PRCOG
Professor of Obstetrics and Gynaecology,
Institute of Obstetrics and Gynaecology,
Queen Charlotte's Hospital for Women,
London

NINA ESSEX, MB, MRCP
Clinical Assistant,
Diabetic Department,
King's College Hospital,
London

LOUISE A. FRIEDMAN, BSc
Research Assistant in Clinical Pharmacology,
Institute of Obstetrics and Gynaecology,
Queen Charlotte's Hospital for Women,
London

D. F. HAWKINS, DSc, FRCOG
Reader in Obstetric Therapeutics,
Institute of Obstetrics and Gynaecology,
Hammersmith Hospital,
London

A. HOPKINS, MD, FRCP
Physician in Charge,
Department of Neurological Sciences,
St Bartholomew's Hospital,
London

ROSALINDE HURLEY, MD, FRCPath
Professor of Microbiology,
Institute of Obstetrics and Gynaecology,
Queen Charlotte's Hospital for Women,
London

**ELIZABETH LETSKY, MB, BS,
  MRCPath**
Consultant Haematologist,
Queen Charlotte's Hospital for Women,
London

vii

LIST OF CONTRIBUTORS

P. J. LEWIS, MD, PhD, MRCP
Senior Lecturer in Clinical Pharmacology,
Institute of Obstetrics and Gynaecology,
Queen Charlotte's Hospital for Women,
London

B. A. LIEBERMAN, MRCOG
Senior Lecturer in Obstetrics and
  Gynaecology,
St Mary's Hospital Medical School,
University of London

S. R. MEADOW, FRCP
Senior Lecturer,
Department of Paediatrics and Child Health,
University of Leeds

HEATHER J. MELLOWS, MB, BS
Resident Medical Officer,
Queen Charlotte's Hospital for Women,
London

I. D. RAMSAY, MD, MRCP, MRCPE
Consultant Physician,
Regional Endocrine Centre,
North Middlesex Hospital,
London

C. W. G. REDMAN, BM, MRCP
Lecturer in Obstetric Medicine,
Department of Obstetrics and Gynaecology,
John Radcliffe Hospital,
Oxford

G. M. STIRRAT, MD, MRCOG
Clinical Reader,
Department of Obstetrics and Gynaecology,
John Radcliffe Hospital,
Oxford

M. de SWIET, MD, MRCP
Consultant Physician,
Queen Charlotte's Hospital for Women,
London

Foreword

The image of obstetrics as a largely manipulative art has changed radically in recent years. The risk to a healthy mother of pregnancy and labour has been markedly reduced and morbidity not mortality is the yardstick by which the quality of maternal care is judged. We are now able to devote far more attention to the fetus whose growth patterns and behaviour *in utero* can be studied in detail by modern and sophisticated technical aids with a resultant improvement in perinatal mortality.

A patient with a pre-existing general disease, however, still presents a problem which is best managed by close co-operation between obstetrician and physician. Essential hypertension, diabetes, heart disease, thyroid disease and epilepsy are examples of disorders which require great care throughout pregnancy and during labour if good maternal and fetal results are to be obtained.

There are many questions still to be answered. What is the place of hypotensive therapy in essential hypertension complicating pregnancy? When should delivery take place in the pregnant diabetic? How should the patient be delivered? What should be her management during labour? What is the risk of fetal abnormality in the epileptic patient who becomes pregnant whilst on anti-epileptic drugs? These questions and others have been the subject of a recent symposium in the Institute of Obstetrics and Gynaecology. The proceedings of that symposium have been brought together and amplified in this volume as an admirable survey of this field which is both a guide to modern therapy and a pointer to developments in the future.

C. J. Dewhurst
President of the Royal College of
Obstetricians and Gynaecologists

Part 1
Hypertension in
Pregnancy

1
The Use of Antihypertensive Drugs in Pregnancy

L. J. BEILIN and C. W. G. REDMAN

Hypertension in pregnancy is generally due to one of two causes, either it is specifically induced by pregnancy, in which case it is always part of a complex disorder (pre-eclampsia, toxaemia) constituting some risk to the fetus; or a woman with pre-existing chronic hypertension may become pregnant. As chronic hypertension predisposes to the development of pre-eclampsia, the two conditions frequently co-exist.

Many mothers with chronic hypertension have pregnancies that are otherwise uncomplicated. The onset of pre-eclampsia is often insidious, whether or not it is preceded by chronic hypertension, and in its early stages is characterized by a rising plasma urate (Redman *et al.*, 1976) and falling platelet count (Redman *et al.*, 1976) (Figure 1.1). The blood-pressure is easily controlled at this stage, but as the condition develops, hypertension becomes more severe and nocturnal hypertension may occur (Redman *et al.*, 1976; Beilin *et al.*, 1974). The glomerular filtration rate declines, proteinuria may appear and the platelet count falls further. The fetus is often small and the mother may cease to gain weight, or alternatively, gain excessively due to fluid retention. The final, and often terminal, stage is augured by oliguria, rapid accumulation of fluid, uncontrollable hypertension, eclamptic fits and death of the fetus and/or mother. This sequence may evolve over a period of weeks or months, but the final phase is often rapid. Thus Figure 1.2 shows an example of how the disorder can progress over a matter of hours, in association with a retroplacental haemorrhage.

The use of antihypertensive drugs has to be considered in the context of this complex and variable natural history of hypertensive pregnancies. The

1

situation is further complicated by the fact that two lives rather than one, are at stake, and that relatively little is known about the aetiology of pre-eclampsia.

WHEN TO USE ANTIHYPERTENSIVE DRUGS IN PREGNANCY

Hypertension with severe pre-eclampsia is of greatest concern when the fetus cannot be safely delivered, i.e. before about the 34th week of pregnancy, for once the fetus has become mature with respect to pulmonary function it is usually safer to deliver the baby rather than prolong the pregnancy.

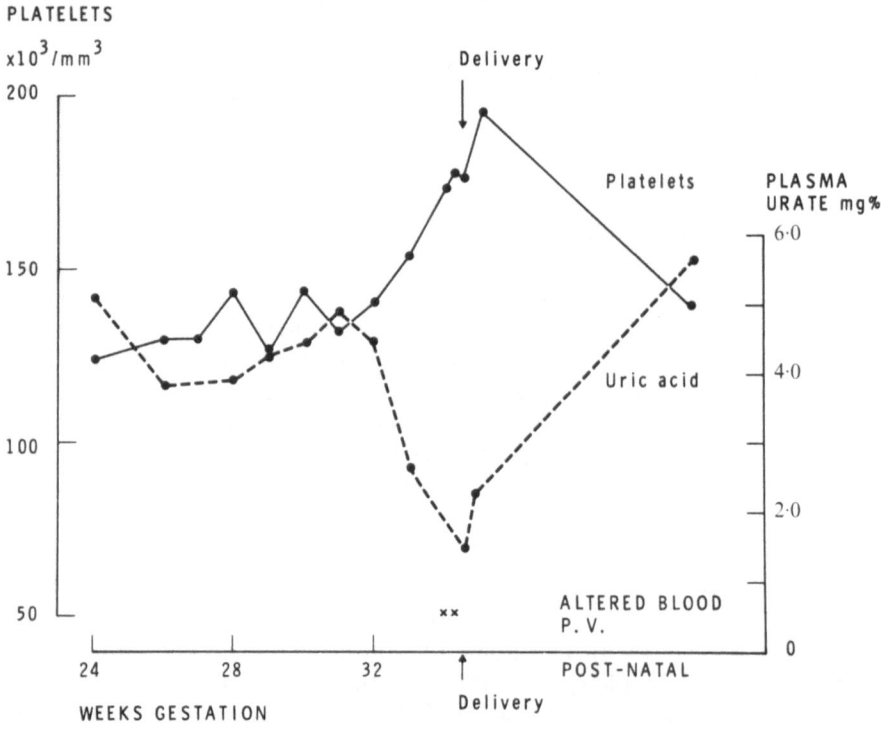

Figure 1.1 27 years old. Parity 1 + 0. Chronic essential hypertension. Blood-pressure rose shortly after uric acid. Proteinuria developed at 35 weeks, just before delivery of 1980 g live infant

Complete bed rest alone is often effective in reducing a moderately elevated blood-pressure in the later stages of pregnancy, and this may be sufficient to carry a patient safely through to delivery. Elective delivery will then lead to a fall in blood-pressure in those with specific hypertension of pregnancy.

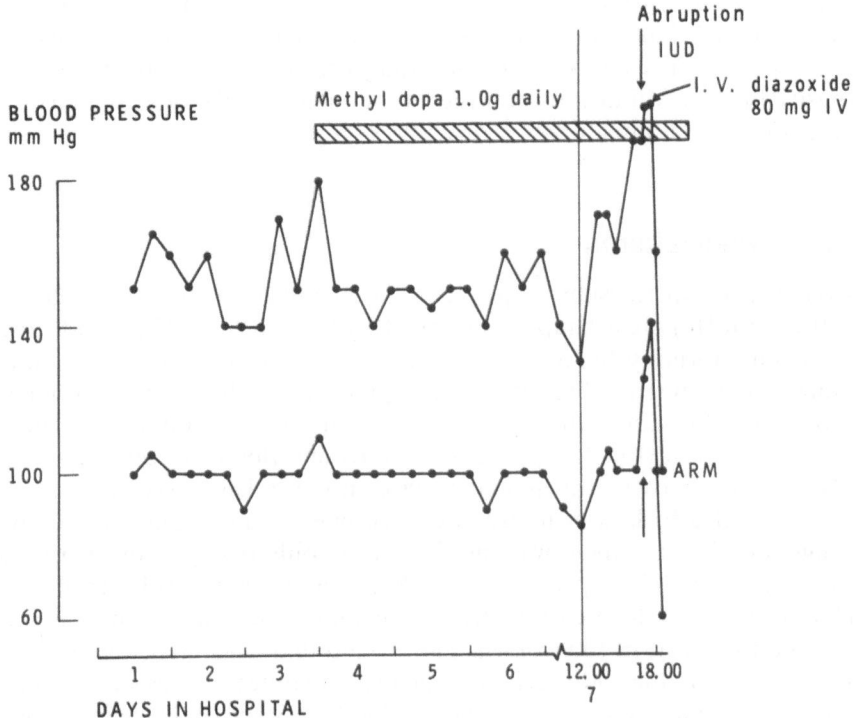

Figure 1.2 28 years old. Parity 0 + 0. Admitted with BP 130/95 mmHg and persistent protein-uria. Infant 1630 g

SEVERE HYPERTENSION

In severe hypertension the pregnant mother is exposed to the same risks as the non-pregnant, namely stroke, left ventricular failure and renal failure, as well as having the specific obstetric risks of eclamptic fits and massive placental haemorrhage.

Kincaid-Smith *et al.* (1966) showed that treatment with methyldopa enabled 32 women with very severe chronic hypertension to be taken through pregnancy with a reasonable perinatal survival. It has also been our experi-ence that drug treatment of severe maternal hypertension enables many pregnancies to continue successfully that would have otherwise been ter-minated on grounds of maternal risk before the fetus was viable. Further-more, provided blood-pressure control is satisfactory, and the pregnancy uncomplicated by pre-eclampsia, then these women can be managed with careful out-patient supervision, rather than being confined to hospital throughout their pregnancies.

Our view has been that the maternal risk from the consequences of hyper-tension are such that specific therapy should be started if pressures exceed

3

170 systolic or 110 mmHg diastolic, despite 24 hours' bed-rest in hospital, or immediately if pressures are above 180/120 mmHg, or if neuroretinopathy, heart failure or symptoms of impending eclampsia develop. Antihypertensive therapy will then protect the mother in all but the most fulminating cases of pre-eclampsia.

MILD HYPERTENSION

Even when hypertension in pregnancy is relatively mild (say 140/90 to 170/110 mmHg) pre-eclampsia is more likely to supervene. Thus the British Perinatal Mortality Survey showed that women with diastolic pressures more than 90 mmHg before 20th week of pregnancy, subsequently developed proteinuria five times more commonly than women with lower blood-pressure in the first half of pregnancy (Butler and Bonham, 1963). The role of antihypertensive treatment in these circumstances has been controversial, and bedevilled by lack of information. Despite the use of antihypertensive drugs for 25 years, there was, until recently, only one controlled trial to assess their value in hypertension in pregnancy. In that trial Leather *et al.* (1968) compared the use of methyldopa combined with a thiazide diuretic, with no treatment in 100 women. They found that when hypertension was recorded before the 20th week of pregnancy, treatment was associated with longer pregnancies and larger babies (Table 1.1). Some of the benefit might

Table 1.1   Early hypertension

	Controls (24)		Treated (23)	
	Present	Absent	Present	Absent
Birthweight (lb. oz.)	4–7	6–1	5–4	6–12
Gestation (weeks)	34	36–3	36–5	38–2

From Leather *et al.* (1968), *Lancet*, i, 488, with permission

have been ascribed to the preparedness of the obstetricians to allow pregnancies to proceed longer when blood-pressure was controlled by treatment. Leather's study also showed fewer mid-pregnancy losses and perinatal deaths in the treated group but the numbers were not large enough to enable definite conclusions to be drawn (Table 1.2).

In Oxford we have carried out a larger controlled trial of antihypertensive therapy, with the hypothesis that if chronic hypertension predisposes to pre-eclampsia by accelerating placental vascular damage, then early blood-pressure reduction might protect the placental circulation, and perhaps retard events leading to pre-eclampsia. It was particularly important to establish whether the use of antihypertensive drugs was safe for the fetus as well as for the mother, and the results of the fetal outcome in this trial show that this is the case (Redman *et al.*, 1976). In brief the trial involved 277 women in whom hypertension was diagnosed if two blood-pressure

Table 1.2 Fetal outcome

Hypertension	Control (48)	Treated (52)
Early	Abortion 3 Perinatal deaths 2	$\left. \begin{matrix} 0 \\ 0 \end{matrix} \right\} < 0\cdot04$
Late	Perinatal deaths 4	6

From Leather *et al.* (1968). *Lancet*, i, 488, with permission

readings taken under standardized conditions using a London School of Hygiene Sphygmomanometer equalled or exceeded 140 mmHg systolic or 90 mmHg diastolic before 28 weeks' gestation, or 150/95 mmHg between 28 and 32 weeks. Thirty of these women were excluded from the trial at the outset for miscellaneous reasons, of which the most important was that the blood-pressure at presentation was too high (> 170/110 mmHg) to with-hold treatment. One hundred and twenty-two women were allocated to treatment with methyldopa and 125 to no treatment.

There were nine fetal/neonatal losses in the control group compared with one in the treated group ($p = 0\cdot013$) (Table 1.3). This difference was mainly due to an increased incidence of mid-pregnancy abortions in control patients. The slight excess of perinatal deaths in the control group was not due to any one pathological cause.

It has been suggested that the blood-pressure reduction in pregnancy might impair placental perfusion and thereby affect fetal growth, development or survival. The mean birthweight of live births was equal in the two groups who entered the trial early, as was the gestation at delivery (Table 1.4).

Table 1.3 Fetal outcome

	Early entry		Late entry	
	Control	Treated	Control	Treated
Allocated to treatment	107	106	18	16
Withdrawn	—	5	—	—
Live births	101	100	15	16
Mid-pregnancy abortions	4	—	—	—
Still births	1	1	2	—
Neonatal deaths	1	—	1	—
Mean duration of treatment (days)	123	114	41	54

Combining early and late entries the total fetal/perinatal losses were 1 in the treated group and 9 in the control group $(p = 0\cdot01)$

From Redman *et al.* (1976). *Lancet*

Table 1.4   Birthweight, placental weight, gestation at delivery

	Early entry		Late entry	
	Control	Treated	Control	Treated
Mean gestation at delivery				
Days ± I.S.D.	267 ± 12*	267 ± 11	264 ± 13†	272 ± 11
Mean birthweight ± I.S.D. kg	3.13 ± 0.5	3.03 ± 0.6	2.69 ± 0.93‡	3.09 ± 0.60
Mean placental weight ± I.S.D. kg	0.59 ± 0.12	0.57 ± 0.13	0.53 ± 0.25	0.61 ± 0.25

Treatment did not significantly affect fetal or placental growth rates

* Excluding 5 mid-trimester miscarriages
† $p < 0.05$
‡ $p > 0.05$

From Redman et al. (1976). Lancet

Moreover, multivariate analysis of factors influencing fetal growth, taking into account gestation at delivery, showed no effect of treatment on birthweight (Tables 1.5 and 1.6).

Table 1.5   Multivariate analysis of factors determining final birthweight

This confirmed no adverse effect of treatment

Equation 1. Dependent variable: birthweight

Maternal factors predicting birthweight	Normalized partial regression coefficient	Significance of linear association
1. Parity	+0.21	<0.01
2. Plasma urate*	−0.28	<0.001
3. Maternal weight*	+0.57	<0.001
4. Urine infection* (0: absent; 1: present)	−0.18	<0.01
5. Cigarettes/day	−0.16	<0.025
6. Haematocrit*	−0.18	<0.01
7. Arm circumference	−0.38	<0.01
8. Plasma sodium*	+0.14	<0.05
9. Increased retinal artery reflex (Scale of 0 to 3)	+0.13	<0.05
Treatment group†	+0.005	Not significant

* Measured at entry of trial
† 0: control; 1: treated

In the trial reported by Leather et al. (1968) treatment was associated with prolonged gestation and increased birthweight. In our study, with careful control over conditions of obstetric intervention, we were unable to show such changes except in the small late-entry group (Table 1.4).

Blood-pressure was significantly reduced in the treated group compared to controls, with the greatest effect in those who had highest pressures initially, and with bigger falls in pressures on standing and after exercise

Table 1.6   Multivariate analysis of factors determining final birthweight

Equation 2. Dependent variable: birthweight adjusted for gestation of delivery and sex of baby

Maternal factors predicting birthweight	Normalized partial regression coefficient	Significance of linear association
1. Cigarettes/day	−0·18	<0·001
2. Haematocrit*	−0·14	<0·01
3. Parity	+0·14	<0·025
4. Plasma urate*	−0·12	<0·025
5. Maternal weight*	+0·23	<0·01
6. Maternal subscapular skin fold*	−0·16	<0·05
Treatment group†	−0·02	Not significant

* Measured at entry to trial
† 0: control; 1: treated

than lying. Treatment largely prevented excessive rise in pressures ante-natally and during labour (Tables 1.7 and 1.8), and 11 of the control patients had to start antihypertensive therapy for severe hypertension (average pressures 182/117 mmHg).

Table 1.7   Maximum blood-pressures: antenatal (early entry group only)

Maximum diastolic	Control group	Treated
⩽89	11	26
90–99	29	46
100–109	29	19
110–119	18	8
⩾120	13	2

$\chi_4^2 = 25\cdot0$; $p < 0\cdot0005$
Treatment prevented excessive pressure rises
Eleven of the controls had to receive treatment because of severe hypertension (group average 182/117 mmHg)

Table 1.8   Maximum blood-pressures during labour

	Control group (% Patients)	Treated	
Maximum systolic (mmHg)			
⩽149	61	80	
150–159	22	13	$\chi_3^2 = 10\cdot63$
160–169	10	3	$p < 0\cdot002$
⩾170	7	4	
Maximum diastolic (mmHg)			
⩽94	50	68	
95–104	29	23	$\chi_3^2 = 21\cdot3$
105–114	16	5	$p < 0\cdot0005$
⩾115	6	3	

Treatment did not affect other features of pre-eclampsia. Proteinuria developed rarely, but with equal frequency in both groups. Serial measurements of plasma urea, uric acid (Table 1.9) and creatinine showed no

Table 1.9 **Maximum antenatal increase in plasma urate**

Urate rise (mg/100 ml)	Early entry		Late entry	
	Control	Treated	Control	Treated
	(Number of patients)		(Number of patients)	
None	6	1	5	5
0·1–1·0	29	29	7	3
1·1–2·0	48	49	3	6
2·1–3·0	17	14	0	2
>3·1	7	8	3	0

differences in renal function throughout pregnancy in treated and control groups. There were no effects of treatment on liver function or bone marrow. One woman developed a positive Coombs test after 26 weeks' treatment, but there was no haemolysis in mother or infant.

Although our trial was organized differently from that of Leather and his colleagues, the results are in many respects comparable and more clear-cut. One similarity was the reduction in mid-pregnancy abortions in the treated group. None occurred in the treated women in either trial. There were too few perinatal deaths to judge the effects of treatment on pre-eclampsia, but in our trial the renal consequences of the disorder occurred to a similar degree in treated and control groups. A raised plasma uric level is an early, sensitive, and invariable indication of pre-eclampsia (Redman et al., 1976), and the fact that the control and treated groups showed similar patterns of change is evidence that the incidence of pre-eclampsia was unaltered by treatment, so this cannot explain the improved outcome in the treated patients.

The apparent beneficial effect of treatment with a methyldopa on the incidence of mid-pregnancy abortions is unexpected, and not obviously related to the antihypertensive action of the drug. The possibility that methyldopa has an alternative pharmacological action accounting for this effect should be entertained. Thus methyldopa might affect the endocrine system of the fetus or mother by an action on the pituitary or hypothalamus. Thus methyldopa increases prolactin secretion in non-pregnant women, although this was not the case in the pregnant women in this trial (Redman et al., 1975). Alternatively methyldopa might indirectly affect uterine tone by altering sympathetic nerve activity to the uterus. Again there is as yet no information on this, but the higher Caesarean section rate following surgical induction in treated women might be relevant.

The condition of the fetus at birth was carefully assessed, and no adverse effects were demonstrated in respect of onset of respiration, 'Apgar' score or duration of stay in hospital. There was, however, a slightly higher incidence of Caesarian section rate in treated mothers following surgical induction of labour. Infants and children are being assessed for subsequent development for up to 7 years by Dr Margaret Ounsted and her colleagues. At 1 year of age there were no signs of any adverse effects of treatment.

We concluded that alpha-methyldopa was relatively safe for mild to moderate chronic hypertension in pregnancy in the context of close and frequent supervision in a specialist unit staffed by physicians and obstetricians. Its use was associated with some fetal benefit which was not obviously ascribable to the prevention of pre-eclampsia.

However, it should be emphasized that other aspects of antenatal care are more important than specific drug therapy in patients with mild hypertension in pregnancy and these are discussed elsewhere (Beilin, 1973; 1974).

THE CHOICE OF ANTIHYPERTENSIVE DRUGS IN PREGNANCY

The choice of drugs for the treatment of hypertension in pregnancy is complicated by the effects of certain drugs on the fetus and on features of pre-eclampsia. In general, drugs are given in the same dosages as for hypertension in women who are not pregnant. Patients with fulminating hypertension or eclampsia present special problems (Beilin, 1973; 1974; Martin, 1974; Joyce and Kenyon, 1972).

Alpha-methyldopa

Alpha-methyldopa reduces blood-pressure by a central action, probably by stimulating alpha receptors in the brain stem, and hence leading to decreased sympathetic outflow from the brain. As has already been mentioned, there are now two controlled trials indicating the relative safety of methyldopa in pregnancy.

In the Oxford study (Redman et al., 1976) daily doses of methyldopa were in the range 0·5–4 g, tending to be higher than those required in non-pregnant subjects (Dollery and Bulpitt, 1973). The average daily dose of methyldopa exceeded 1 g at all gestations and rose with advancing pregnancy to a maximum of 1·7 g daily. Later in pregnancy greater use of other drugs was necessary for effective blood-pressure control, and the most useful adjunct to methyldopa was hydrallazine (100–300 mg daily) which was used in 12 of the patients treated in the trial. Depression was not a problem when the drug was avoided in patients with a history of this disorder. Systematic enquiry revealed that drowsiness and faintness on standing were the only symptoms occurring in significant excess in treated patients (Table 1.10).

Table 1.10   Symptoms recorded antenatally (early entry group)

	Control group (107)	Treated group (101)	χ_1^2 p
Impaired appetite	34	30	NS
Impaired sleep	67	73	NS
Reduced energy	69	85	<0·01
Depression	60	59	
Dizziness	49	63	<0·02
Headaches Vomiting Bowel disturbance	No differences		

Seventeen patients in the trial stopped methyldopa, often from multiple complaints, of which the commonest was lethargy. Of the three major psychiatric episodes in the study requiring in-patient treatment two involved control patients, and the third was a woman discharged post-natally on methyldopa. The finding of only one case of a positive Coombs test out of over 100 treated patients probably reflects the fact that the average duration of treatment in the trial was 18 weeks, and that in the non-pregnant it is unusual for a Coombs test to become positive before 6 months of treatment.

Hydrallazine

This drug acts directly on vascular smooth muscle as a non-specific vaso-dilator. It has been extensively used for hypertensive emergencies in pregnancy (Riva, 1956), but is effective orally when combined with drugs acting on the sympathetic nervous system which block the reflex increase in cardiac output that occurs when the blood-pressure falls as a result of peripheral vasodilatation. In the non-pregnant, the long-term use of hydrallazine in high doses is often associated with the appearance of antinuclear antibodies and a syndrome resembling disseminated lupus erythematosis. This is unlikely to be a problem when the drug is used for relatively short periods in pregnancy at doses below 300 mg/day. Thus, hydrallazine may be combined usefully with oral methyldopa, clonidine, debrisoquine or bethanidine, starting at a dose of 25 mg given three or four times daily. Fluid retention is more likely to be a problem when these two types of drugs are combined, but in our practice it has never been enough to warrant diuretic therapy except in patients with eclampsia and oliguric renal failure. Flushing, palpitations, throbbing headaches and vomiting are common when hydrallazine is given intravenously or intramuscularly. The use of hydrallazine with drugs acting on the sympathetic nervous system has the theoretical attraction of maintaining cardiac output and renal blood-flow, despite reduction in blood-pressure.

Clonidine

Clonidine, like methyldopa, reduces blood-pressure by a central mechanism, stimulating alpha receptors in the brain stem. The blood-pressure reduction is quantitatively and qualitatively similar, sedation is common and depression may occur. Dryness of the mouth is more troublesome, and sudden cessation of clonidine in the non-pregnant has been characterized by very severe 'rebound' hypertension due to sudden discharge of catecholamines into the circulation. For these reasons there appear to be no advantages, and possibly some hazard, in using this drug in pregnancy as an alternative to methyldopa.

Sympathetic neurone blocking agents

Debrisoquine (Athanassiades *et al.*, 1966), bethanidine and guanethidine interfere with the release of noradrenaline from the peripheral sympathetic nerve ending, and all reduce blood-pressures in pregnancy. Postural hypotension is possibly even more troublesome than in the non-pregnant. In the absence of autoregulation of the placental circulation this increases the theoretical risk of impaired placental perfusion with these drugs. Guanethidine is least well tolerated due to excessive diarrhoea and its prolonged action. We have found debrisoquine a satisfactory alternative to methyldopa where the latter was contraindicated by a history of depression or by other side effects.

Reserpine

Reserpine and other rauwolfia alkaloids are centrally acting hypotensive agents which were successfully used to treat severe hypertension in pregnancy before more satisfactory drugs became available (Landesman *et al.*, 1957). However, they cause nasal obstruction in the newborn and have adverse effects on the infants' respiration and temperature regulation (Desmond *et al.*, 1957; Anagnostakis and Matsaniotis, 1974); moreover, mothers receiving them are prone to puerperal depression. Their effects can last for several weeks due to generalized depletion of tissue catecholamines, and they should therefore no longer be used in pregnancy.

Diuretics

The available evidence indicates that the only situations in which diuretics should be used in pregnancy are for the treatment of heart failure, and to see whether the kidneys are capable of excreting urine in women with eclampsia and severe oliguria. Oedema *per se* does no harm providing it is not in the lungs or brain.

There are several reasons why diuretic drugs are contraindicated in most pregnancies. First and foremost there is no evidence that they are of value — several well-controlled trials (Table 1.11) have shown no benefit from their

Table 1.11   Diuretics in pregnancy—satisfactory trials

		No. of patients	Benefit claimed
Weseley and Douglas	1962	267	None
Flowers et al.	1962	519	None
Kraus et al.	1966	1,030	None
Tervila and Vartiainen	1971	211	None

use in the prophylaxis or treatment of pre-eclampsia. The results of the largest of these are summarized in Table 1.12 (Kraus et al., 1966).

Table 1.12   Diuretics in pregnancy

Treatment had no effect on:	Placebo (506)	Hydrochlorthiazide (524)
1. Fetal growth		
2. Fetal loss	3·0%	3·8%
3. 'Pre-eclampsia'	2·7%	3·0%
4. All hypertension	19·6%	21·8%

From Kraus et al. (1966). J. Am. Med. Assoc., 198, 115c, with permission

Trials from which some benefits have been claimed from the use of diuretics in pregnancy have all been unsatisfactory (Table 1.13). The trial by Finnerty and Bepko (1966) is the most important of these, in that its results are still widely accepted. Table 1.14 summarizes the main features of this study, which appeared to show an outstanding effect of diuretic therapy in converting a perinatal mortality of 5% in the control group to 0·7% in the treated group. However, patients who received diuretic therapy were managed differently from those who did not, in terms of investigation and follow up. Thus urines were examined for bacteriuria in the treated patients but not in the controls, and patients with bacteriuria were excluded from the study. This alone could be of crucial importance in view of the strong

Table 1.13   Diuretics in pregnancy—unsatisfactory trials

		No. of patients	Benefit claimed
Cuadros and Tatum	1964	1771	Yes
Menzies	1964	100	Yes
Fallis et al.	1964	78	Yes
Finnerty and Bepko	1966	3083	Yes

association between asymptomatic bacteriuria, premature labour, abortion and perinatal mortality (Kass, 1962; Wren, 1969). It is not clear, moreover, from Finnerty and Bepko's study precisely when the bacteriuric patients were excluded from the trial. The second major criticism of their study arises from the fact that 201 of their treated group who were found not to be taking drugs satisfactorily, were transferred to the control group. It is well known that a poor outcome in pregnancy is strongly associated with failure to comply with antenatal care. Thus the patients in the control group were boosted by an unknown number with asymptomatic bacteriuria, and a further 13% who complied poorly with therapy, whilst the treated group were shorn of these high-risk patients at various stages during the study. The difference in fetal outcome between treated and control groups can probably be accounted for by the bias introduced, rather than by any specific effect of treatment.

The second reason for not wishing to use diuretics in pregnancy is that they raise serum uric acid and urea levels, thus obscuring interpretation of tests, which at an early stage of pregnancy are of considerable value in predicting the development of severe pre-eclampsia and fetal death (Redman *et al.*, 1976). The third reason for avoiding diuretic therapy in pregnancy is that it may do harm. Thiazide induced pancreatitis has also been described. Hypokalaemia is common, although only severe in a minority of cases (Tervila and Vartiainen, 1971).

Women with severe pre-eclampsia have a low cardiac output (Littler *et al.*, 1973) and reduced plasma volume despite the generalized fluid retention, so that the chances of a further reduction in cardiac output and reduced placental perfusion with diuretic therapy is more likely than not in

Table 1.14 'Controlled' trial of diuretics in pregnancy

	'Treated'	'Control'
Initial 'selection'	1541	1542
Bacteriuria (prior exclusion)	? 5–22%	Not sought
Poor compliance	201 transferred	Unknown
Final numbers	1340	1743
Perinatal mortality	0·7%	5%

From Finnerty and Bepko (1966). *J. Am. Med. Assoc.*, **195**, 429

this situation. Occasional cases of severe fluid and electrolyte depletion with collapse have been reported (Palomaki and Lindheimer, 1970). The uses and abuses of diuretics in pregnancy have been reviewed by Lindheimer and Katz (1974), Pitkin *et al.* (1972) and Gray (1968). There have also been anecdotal reports of neonatal thrombocytopenia (Finnerty and Assali, 1964; Rodriguez *et al.*, 1964), jaundice (Crossland and Flowers, 1963) and neonatal haemolysis (Harley, 1964).

Finally, it was our impression when we used diuretics in pregnancy that they were less effective at potentiating the action of antihypertensive drugs than in the non-pregnant. '

Beta-adrenergic blockade

There is little published on the use of beta receptor antagonists in hypertensive pregnancies. Anecdotal reports have suggested harm from interference with uterine tone and contractions (Barnes, 1970). Intravenous practolol blocks the relaxing effect of salbutamol infusion on uterine tone, and causes fetal as well as maternal bradycardia (McDevitt et al., 1975). There are also a number of brief accounts (reported elsewhere in this symposium) of propranolol causing beta blockade in the fetus in pregnant animals, and in particular, impaired survival of fetuses subjected to uterine ischaemia in primates. Given that all the beta blockers currently available reduce maternal cardiac output, and the experimental data suggesting that the ability of the fetus to survive a compromised uterine circulation is impaired in the presence of beta blockade, it is doubtful whether large-scale studies of the use of beta blockers in hypertensive pregnancy are justified, unless agents are developed which do not cross the placenta in an active form. Goodwin has described the successful supervision of 18 patients with hypertrophic cardiomyopathy treated with propranolol or practolol. However, the doses used in this study were fairly low (Turner et al., 1968) and the situation cannot be compared with that of severe pre-eclampsia where fetal bradycardia is often a sign of impending intrauterine death. At present there seems little reason for using beta blockers in pregnancy unless the patient with severe hypertension is intolerant of the other drugs referred to above.

OTHER MEASURES

Oral diazoxide will sometimes reduce blood-pressure when other drugs have failed (Pohl et al., 1972) but the drug delays fetal bone growth and leads to alopecia in the newborn (Milner and Chouskey, 1972), as well as causing excessive fluid retention and diabetes mellitus in the mother.

Sedatives and tranquilizing drugs have little or no antihypertensive effect unless given in near anaesthetic doses, and usually lull the doctor into a false sense of security. Their use should be reserved for treating symptoms of anxiety per se.

Anecdotal reports of the successful use of various drugs and measures to treat hypertension in pregnancy continue to punctuate the literature. These uncontrolled reports are usually misleading, particularly as the majority of women with chronic maternal hypertension have a successful outcome to their pregnancies without drug treatment, a substantial proportion of women with pre-eclampsia will do likewise, and many with severe complications in previous pregnancies will not show these subsequently.

CONCLUSIONS

The use of drugs to treat hypertension in pregnancy must still be considered primarily from the point of view of preventing the maternal consequences of severe hypertension. In two controlled trials the use of methyldopa for the treatment of mild to moderate hypertension in pregnancy has been associated with an improved fetal outcome, largely due to a reduced incidence of mid-trimester abortions. Such treatment appears to be relatively safe in the context of close supervision by physician and obstetrician in a specialist antenatal clinic. There is no evidence that treating hypertension influences the progression of the underlying disorder in pre-eclampsia. However, treatment of severe hypertension will help protect the mothers and thereby enable many pregnancies to be continued that otherwise would be terminated on the grounds of maternal risk.

References

Anagnostakis, D. and Matsaniotis, N. (1974). Neonatal cold injury and maternal reserpine administration. *Lancet*, **ii**, 471

Athanassiadis, D., Cranston, W. I., Juel-Jensen, B. E. and Oliver, D. O. (1966). Clinical observations on the effects of debrisoquine sulphate in patients with high blood-pressure. *Br. Med. J.*, **2**, 732

Barden, T. P. and Strander, R. W. (1968). Effects of adrenergic blocking agents and catecholamines in human pregnancy. *Am. J. Obstet. Gynecol.*, **102**, 226

Barnes, A. B. (1970). Chronic propranolol administration during pregnancy. *J. Reprod. Med.*, **5**, 79

Beilin, L. J. (1973). Hypertension in pregnancy. Parts I and II. *Teach-In*, **2**, 451; **2**, 489

Beilin, L. J. (1974). The treatment of hypertension during pregnancy. *Prescribers J.*, **14**, 125

Beilin, L. J., Redman, C. W. G. and Bonnar, J. (1974). Hypertension in pregnancy. In J. G. G. Ledingham (ed.) *10th Advanced Medicine Symposium*, pp. 3–19 (London: Pitman Medical)

Butler, N. R. and Alberman, E. D. (eds.) (1969). *Perinatal Problems.* The second report of the 1958 British Perinatal Mortality Survey (Edinburgh: E. & S. Livingstone)

Butler, N. R. and Bonham, D. G. (eds.) (1963). *Perinatal Mortality.* The first report of the 1958 British Perinatal Mortality Survey (Edinburgh: E. & S. Livingstone)

Crossland, D. and Flowers, C. (1963). Chlorothiazide and its relationship to neonatal jaundice. *Obstet. Gynecol.*, **22**, 500

Cuadros, A. and Tatum, H. J. (1964). The prophylactic and therapeutic use of bendroflumethiazide in pregnancy. *Am. J. Obstet. Gynecol.*, **89**, 891

Desmond, M. M., Rogers, S. F., Lindley, J. E. and Moyer, J. H. (1957). Management of toxaemia of pregnancy with reserpine; II, The newborn infant. *Obstet. Gynecol.*, **10**, 140

Dollery, C. T. and Bulpitt, C. J. (1973). *Hypertension Mechanisms and Management*, p. 299 (New York: Grane and Stratton)

Fallis, N. E., Planche, W. C., Mosey, L. M. and Langford, H. G. (1964). Thiazide versus placebo in prophylaxis of toxaemia of pregnancy in primigravid patients. *Am. J. Obstet. Gynecol.*, **88**, 502

Finnerty, F. A., Jr. and Assali, N. S. (1964). Thiazide and neonatal thrombocytopenia. *N. Engl. J. Med.*, **271**, 160

Finnerty, F. A. and Bepko, F. J. (1966). Lowering the perinatal mortality and the prematurity rate. *J. Am. Med. Assoc.*, **195**, 429

Goodwin, J. F. (1973). Treatment of the cardiomyopathies. *Am. J. Cardiol.*, **32**, 341

Gray, M. J. (1968). Use and abuse of thiazides in pregnancy. *Clin. Obst. Gynecol.*, **11**, 568

Hans, S. F. and Kopelman, H. (1964). Methyldopa in treatment of severe toxaemia of pregnancy. *Br. Med. J.*, **1**, 736

Harley, J. D. (1964). Thiazide induced neonatal haemolysis. *Br. Med. J.*, **1**, 696

Joyce, D. N. and Kenyon, V. G. (1972). The use of diazepam and hydrallazine in the treatment of severe pre-eclampsia. *J. Obstet. Gynaecol. Br. Commonw.*, **79**, 250

Kass, E. H. (1962). Pyelonephritis and bacteriuria. *Ann. Intern. Med.*, **56**, 46

Kincaid-Smith, P., Bullen, H. and Mills, J. (1966). Prolonged use of methyldopa in severe hypertension in pregnancy. *Br. Med. J.*, **1**, 274

Kraus, G. W., Marchese, J. R. and Yen, S. (1966). Prophylactic use of hydrochlorothiazide in pregnancy. *J. Am. Med. Assoc.*, **198**, 1150

Landesman, R., McLarn, W. D., Ollstein, R. N. and Mendlesohn, B. (1957). Reserpine in toxaemia of pregnancy. *Obstet Gynecol.*, **9**, 377

Leather, H. M., Humphreys, D. M., Baker, P. B. and Chadd, M. A. (1968). A controlled trial of hypotensive agents in hypertension in pregnancy. *Lancet*, **i**, 488

Lindheimer, M. D. and Katz, A. I. (1974). Sodium and diuretics in pregnancy. *Obstet Gynecol.*, **44**, 434

Littler, W. A., Redman, C. W. G., Bonnar, J., Beilin, L. J. and Lee, G. de J. (1973). Reduced pulmonary arterial compliance in hypertensive pregnancy. *Lancet*, **i**, 1274

McDevitt, D. G., Wallace, R. J., Roberts, A. and Whitfield, C. R. (1975). The uterine and cardiovascular effects of salbutamol and practolol during labour. *Br. J. Obstet. Gynaecol.*, **82**, 442

Mahon, W. A., Reid, D. W. J. and Day, R. A. (1967). The in vivo effects of beta-adrenergic stimulation and blockade on the human uterus at term. *J. Pharmacol. Exp. Ther.*, **156**, 178

Martin, J. D. (1974). A critical survey of drugs used in the treatment of hypertensive crises of pregnancy. *Med. J. Aust.*, **2**, 252

Menzies, D. N. (1964). Controlled trial of chlorothiazide in treatment of early pre-eclampsia. *Br. Med. J.*, **1**, 739

Milner, R. D. G. and Chouskey, S. K. (1972). Effects of fetal exposure to diazoxide in man. *Arch. Dis. Child.*, **47**, 537

Palomaki, J. F. and Lindheimer, M. D. (1970). Sodium depletion simulating deterioration in a toxaemic pregnancy. *N. Engl. J. Med.*, **282**, 88

Pitkin, R. M., Kaminetzky, H. A. and Newton, M. (1972). Maternal nutrition: a selective review of clinical topics. *Obstet. Gynecol.*, **40**, 773

Pohl, J. E. F., Thurston, H., Davis, D. and Morgan, M. Y. (1972). Successful use of oral diazoxide in the treatment of severe toxaemia of pregnancy. *Br. Med. J.*, **2**, 568

Redman, C. W. G., Beilin, L. J. and Bonnar, J. (1976). A trial of antihypertensive treatment in pregnancy—blood-pressure control and side effects. (In press)

Redman, C. W. G., Beilin, L. J. and Bonnar, J. (1976). Renal function in pre-eclampsia. In Rosalinde Hurley (ed.) *The Pathology of Pregnancy, J. Clin. Pathol.*, **29**, *Suppl. (R. Coll. Pathol.)*, **10**, pp. 91–94

Redman, C. W. G., Beilin, L. J. and Bonnar, J. (1976). Variability of blood-pressure in normal and abnormal pregnancy. *Cli. Sci. & Mol. Med. Suppl. on Hypertension.* (In press)

Redman, C. W. G., Bonnar, J., Beilin, L. J. and McNeilly, A. S. (1975). Prolactin in hypertensive pregnancy. *Br. Med. J.*, **1**, 304

Redman, C. W. G., Beilin, L. J., Bonnar, J. and Ounsted, M. K. (1976). Fetal outcome in trial of antihypertensive treatment in pregnancy. *Lancet*, **ii**, 753

Riva, H. L. (1956). Experiences with apresoline in toxaemia of pregnancy and hypertension. *Am. J. Obstet. Gynecol.*, **72**, 48

Rodriguez, S. U., Leikin, S. L. and Hiller, M. C. (1964). Neonatal thrombocytopenia associated with antepartum administration of thiazide drugs. *N. Engl. J. Med.*, **270**, 881

Rogers, S. F., Lindley, J. E., Moyer, J. H. and Desmond, M. M. (1957). Management of toxaemia of pregnancy with reserpine. *Obstet. Gynecol.*, **10**, 17

Smith, R. W. and Yarborough, C. J. (1967). Plasma volume prediction in pregnancy. *Am. J. Obstet. Gynecol.*, **99**, 18

Tervila, L. and Vartiainen, E. (1971). The effects and side effects of diuretics in the prophylaxis of toxaemia of pregnancy. *Acta Obstet. Gynaecol. Scand.*, **50**, 351

Turner, G. M., Oakley, C. M. and Dixon, H. G. (1968). Management of pregnancy complicated by hypertrophic obstructive cardiomyopathy. **4**, 281

Weseley, A. C. and Douglas, G. N. (1962). Continuous use of chlorothiazide for prevention of toxaemia of pregnancy. *Obstet. Gynecol.*, **19**, 355

Wren, B. C. (1969). Subclinical urinary infection in pregnancy. *Med. J. Austr.*, **24**, 1220

Discussion

Wright, N., London: Did you divide your patients into primigravid and multiparous patients and have you taken into account their age and previous obstetric history?

Beilin: The control and treated groups were similar in all of those respects.

Redman, T. F., Leeds: What was your dosage regimen of methyldopa?

Beilin: We gave the methyldopa four times a day.

Redman: Do you think this frequency administration is really necessary? Surely you would have much better patient compliance administering the drug once or twice a day?

Beilin: We have not studied whether methyldopa given twice a day would have been as effective as four times a day. It was our impression that some patients required dosage four times daily in order to produce good blood-pressure control. I agree patient compliance would probably be better if we could use a twice daily regimen.

2
Antihypertensive Drugs and Uterine Blood Flow

D. F. HAWKINS

A systolic blood-pressure of 135 mmHg or more, or a diastolic blood-pressure of 85 mmHg or more is abnormal in pregnancy. If an elevated blood-pressure is recorded before 20 weeks maturity, the condition is usually termed essential hypertension in pregnancy. The majority of such patients will have latent or mild benign essential hypertension, brought to light by the sharp discrimination of the abnormal blood-pressure which pregnancy engenders. Some are established hypertensives. The remainder have general disorders such as renal disease, aortic regurgitation, congenital heart disease, thyrotoxicosis, systemic lupus erythematosus or a simple anxiety state. Fortunately, after the primary condition has been treated adequately, the management of any residual hypertension is the same as that of the commoner types of hypertension in pregnancy.

Some patients will have some proteinuria at the start of pregnancy, signifying renal involvement; the most severe cases may have a degree of nitrogen retention with a raised blood urea. Deterioration in the hypertension during the pregnancy may be accompanied by development or exacerbation of proteinuria or nitrogen retention. Little clinical purpose is served by trying to distinguish some or all these patients as having 'superimposed toxaemia' — the hypertension and its consequences are getting worse and require appropriate management. Sudden development of oedema in essential hypertension in pregnancy can signify deterioration with a fetus at considerable risk.

The definition of pre-eclampsia as 'hypertension coming on late in pregnancy, whether or not accompanied by albuminuria or oedema', is more appropriate to current practice than the classical triad. Today, most patients with pre-eclampsia are treated and delivered before they ever develop

19

proteinuria. Oedema alone conveys no increased hazard to the fetus. In conjunction with the other signs of pre-eclampsia it may confirm the severity of the situation. Development of finger or facial oedema signifies a generalized retention of fluid and electrolytes in the extracellular space.

The term 'fulminating pre-eclampsia' is useful, signifying rapid development of serious hypertension in late pregnancy, perhaps with albuminuria and oedema, with consequent risk to mother and fetus.

PATHOLOGY

Hypertension developing in pregnancy or exacerbation of pre-existing hypertension is in general, at least initially, vasospastic in nature, with increased peripheral resistance. The hazards to the mother include the pathology of continued hypertension and of any degree of renal involvement, perhaps persisting after the pregnancy. Severe exacerbations of hypertension can result in eclampsia, cerebral vascular accidents, hypertensive encephalopathy, cerebral oedema, left ventricular failure, liver damage or renal failure.

The adverse effects of hypertension in pregnancy on the fetus are generally believed to be mediated by effects on the placental circulation. It is well established in animal experiments (Wigglesworth, 1964) and less well in humans (Theobald, 1961) that restriction of the uterine circulation can lead to intrauterine growth retardation or to intrauterine death of the fetus. In humans, the fetus may be affected by impairment of the maternal blood-supply to the placenta, or by restriction of the placental circulation consequent on intervillous fibrin deposition or infarction. The blood-supply may be restricted by reduced flow through the uterine artery, and by hyperplastic arteriosclerotic changes which develop in the arteries supplying the chorio-decidual lakes (Robertson et al., 1967). These degenerative arterial changes may be established by the beginning of the third trimester in essential hypertension; the acute atherosis due to pre-eclampsia occurs somewhat later. Chronic impairment of the placental blood-supply leads to placental insufficiency, intrauterine growth retardation and a dysmature baby, with the risk of antepartum, intrapartum or neonatal death of the fetus. More acute reduction in placental blood-supply, or exacerbation of chronic insufficiency, perhaps by the added restrictions on chorio-decidual flow caused by the myometrial contractions of labour, may produce fetal distress.

HAEMODYNAMICS

The blood-supply to the placental bed may be considered schematically as in Figure 2.1; the uterine artery supplies both the myometrium and the chorio-decidual lakes.

It follows that:

(a) Hypertension due to an overall increase in peripheral resistance which includes vasoconstriction in the uterine artery or the branches supplying the placenta will tend to reduce placental blood flow. If intravascular volume is

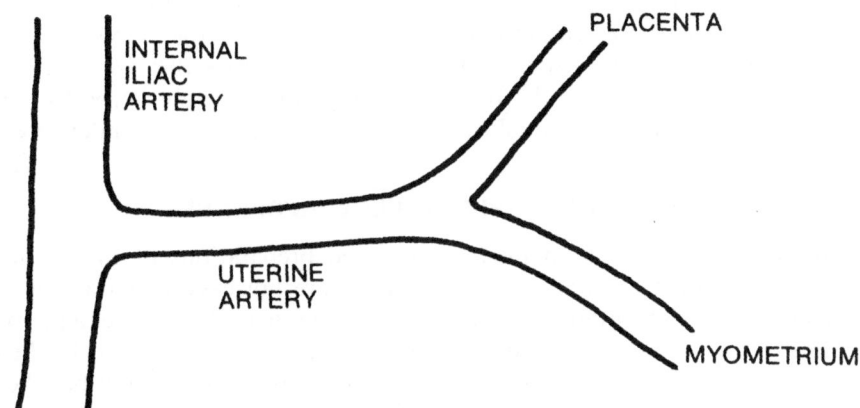

Figure 2.1 Schematic representation of the maternal blood-supply to the placenta

constant there must be compensatory vasodilatation elsewhere, but in moderate to severe hypertension in pregnancy there is often haemoconcentration and reduced intravascular volume (Liley, 1970), perhaps due to increased transudation of fluid into the extravascular compartments. In this condition there can be chronic reduction of uterine blood flow without constriction elsewhere.

(b) Reduction of such hypertension by an agent which relaxes the vasospasm in the utero-placental circulation as part of its mode of action will then improve the uterine blood flow.

(c) Reduction of hypertension by an agent which does not relieve uteroplacental vasospasm or to a level below that compatible with the degree to which the utero-placental vessels relax will cause diminished pressure in the uterine artery and a reduction in uterine blood flow.

(d) If the flow through the uterine artery is constant, an agent which causes vasodilatation in the myometrial circulation but not in the placental supply will cause a reduction in chorio-decidual blood flow, the flow being partly diverted to the myometrium. Such an agent can only be of value to the placenta if it enhances flow through the uterine artery to a point which over-compensates the increased myometrial flow.

(e) If the sclerotic change in the chorio-decidual vessels of the placental bed has proceeded to a point where they are incapable of dilatation, then reduction in the systemic blood-pressure will cause a reduction in flow through them. Therapy in essential hypertension must therefore aim at controlling blood-pressure before the vessels become rigid, in the hope that the damage will thereby be limited.

(f) In a hypertensive situation where a relatively rapid rise in blood-pressure occurs within at most a day or two or in labour, it is likely to have been caused by vasospasm rather than structural change in the vessels. It is then reasonable to use symptomatic measures to control the blood-pressure to a level of the same order as that pertaining before the rise. If more energetic therapy reduces the blood-pressure to completely normal levels this may reduce uterine blood flow to a point where the fetus is endangered.

ASSESSMENT OF UTERINE BLOOD FLOW RESPONSES

Considerable use has been made of isolated preparations of the uterine artery to examine responses to drugs. They are not easy preparations to handle and their sensitivity and responses to drugs may change over a period of hours. The usual sources are animals or non-pregnant women. In their acutely denervated state the responses of these preparations cannot be taken to represent those of the uterine artery *in situ* in a pregnant woman. Their only value is to examine pharmacodynamic interactions when a response, clearly established to occur *in vivo*, can be reliably demonstrated in the isolated artery. Little attempt seems to have been made to differentiate myometrial and placental components of the uterine circulation under isolated conditions.

Myometrial autografts in pregnant rabbit ear chambers (Cliff *et al.*, 1963) are an elegant preparation for the study of responses to drugs of the myometrial vasculature. The reactions observed do not necessarily parallel those of the placental bed vessels.

Animals have been widely used in acute experiments to examine responses of the uterine circulation to pharmacological agents. Flowmeters based on electro-magnetic or ultrasonic principles can be implanted chronically and studies of uterine blood flow made over a period of days in conscious experimental animals such as sheep, goats, dogs, rhesus monkeys or baboons. The uterine circulations and their innervation in these species differ somewhat from those in the human. Allowing for species differences in drug responses, it is only possible to extrapolate general principles to the situation in the human female. For example, much basic work has been performed using sheep, but in this animal the vascular resistance of the placenta is only about 20% of that in humans and placental blood flow is about four times that in the human (Bruce and Abdul-Karim, 1974). In sheep the uterine blood flow can be reduced very considerably without evoking signs of fetal distress (Greiss, 1967). The other major problem with animal work is the absence of the very disease patterns in pregnancy with which we are concerned—essential hypertension and pre-eclampsia. Twin lambing disease in sheep has some points of similarity with human pregnancy toxaemia but the analogy is not close enough to be of real value.

In pregnant women, technical difficulties in the measurement of uterine blood flow are considerable; most methods allow a single measurement only. This means that attempts to assess drug and other effects involve statistical comparisons between series of patients in which uncontrolled variables mask the response.

The Fick principle employing nitrous oxide has been used to make single assessments of total uterine blood flow at term in women undergoing Caesarean hysterectomy—an operation for sterilization which is rarely considered to be justified in Great Britain. It is well established that the flow is of the order of 450 ml/min, with a range from 250 to 850 ml/min, correspondinto to 80–150 ml/min/kg of uterus and its contents (Blechner et al., 1974; Greiss, 1974; and earlier workers cited therein).

Angiographic procedures have been used to make 'before and after' comparisons (Theobald, 1961). It is possible not only to measure the size of individual blood-vessels but also to assess blood flow by the rate of disappearance of the radio-opaque dye (Bienarz et al., 1969). Application of serial angiograms is strictly limited, since the arterial puncture required is an invasive procedure which is not free from risk and radiation exposure is involved.

Since the injection of radioactive sodium into the chorio-decidual space was used by Browne and Veall (1953) to provide the first convincing evidence that maternal placental blood flow was reduced in essential hypertension and pre-eclampsia, use has been made of clearance techniques. Single measurements which might have had clinical value were perhaps justifiable, but there is now a reasonable reluctance to invade the placenta with a needle or use radioactive agents. The inhalation of xenon-133, followed by monitoring of the placental site and expired air (Jacoby et al., 1972) is much safer, with lower radiation exposure. Even with a sophisticated computer analysis, the method was insufficiently accurate to demonstrate differences in flow between normal and hypertensive pregnancies, though three of the four women who produced dysmature babies were found to have diminished clearance from the placental site.

Myometrial blood flow can be estimated in pregnant women by the clearance of radioactive substances injected into the myometrium (Morris et al., 1955), but there is again reluctance to perform more than a single observation or a 'before and after' assessment in any one patient. Myometrial flow does not necessarily correlate with that through the maternal placenta. Dixon et al. (1963) and Cox et al. (1963) did not find the same degree of association between hypertension and myometrial blood flow as was found with maternal placental blood flow.

Prill and Götz (1961) described the use of a 'thermistor' needle probe inserted into the substance of the cervix to measure uterine blood flow. The probe contains a small heating element and a thermocouple enabling blood flow to be monitored in terms of rate of heat dissipation. It is inserted laterally in the cervix so that its tip lies near the branches of the uterine artery and the acute effect of drugs administered to the mother can be observed (Brotánek and Hodr, 1967). Disadvantages are that the method is invasive, that only qualitative observations can be made, and that the records probably reflect myometrial blood flow rather than that through the placenta.

The final arbiter of the adequacy of uterine blood flow is the outcome with respect to the baby. Intrauterine growth retardation and the production of a dysmature baby may be taken to reflect chronically insufficient placental blood flow. Babies, whether stillborn or healthy, can be assessed against 'weight for dates' charts and categorized by the population percentile in which they fall. The procedure can be criticized in that it involves compounding three errors—the population variation, the sample error in preparation of the curves and the sample error of the cases studied—but it is at least definitive and the data is readily obtained. Acute inadequacy of the placental circulation, for example in labour, may be assessed by the occurrence of the clinical parameters of fetal distress, by fetal blood gas sampling, and by the state of the baby at birth.

In summary, the methods available for assessing the response of uterine blood flow to drugs in the pregnant woman are seriously limited by the difficulty of safe access to the utero-placental circulation, the difficulty of securing repeated observations over a period of time, the problem of distinguishing responses of the maternal placental vasculature from those of the myometrial vessels and the statistical difficulties introduced by uncontrollable variables. In consequence, much of the information we have on the effects of drugs on blood flow to the human pregnant uterus has the insecure basis of extrapolation and analogy from situations of dubious comparability.

ANTIHYPERTENSIVE THERAPY

The purposes of antihypertensive therapy in pregnancy are to protect the mother against the consequences of continued hypertension and those of acute exacerbations, and to protect the placental blood flow from the vascular damage believed to result from chronic maternal hypertension and from the acute impairment associated with a rapid increase in blood-pressure.

The apparent effectiveness of treatment in achieving these objectives is influenced by the attitudes of the obstetricians and physicians concerned. In some centres the reaction to pregnancy in a patient with essential hypertension is to advise termination of the pregnancy and sterilization. In others, this situation is regarded in the same light as pregnancy in a woman with diabetes or heart disease who wants a baby. There is a small risk to the mother and an increased risk of a perinatal loss. At Hammersmith Hospital, with a very wide experience in the use of hypotensive drugs for the last 25 years, hypertensive women who want a pregnancy are referred to the obstetric department as a matter of routine and the great majority achieve a healthy baby without any deterioration in maternal condition.

It is well established that the essential hypertensive mother can be protected by controlling her blood-pressure with drugs. With the correct use of hypotensive agents, alone or in combination, it should be extremely rare that essential hypertension becomes uncontrolled to a degree where termination of the pregnancy has to be contemplated before the baby is viable. It is equally clear that little benefit to the fetus is conferred by the exhibition of hypotensive drugs late in pregnancy. Carey (1959) showed that use of protoveratrine in the third trimester did not improve fetal prognosis and Morris (1953) obtained the same result using hexamethonium. This is probably because the arteriosclerotic changes in the placental vessels are established by the third trimester and reduction of blood-pressure in an essential hypertensive does not then improve flow and may reduce it (Dixon et al., 1963). It is therefore desirable in essential hypertension that blood-pressure should be controlled from early on in pregnancy. Patients whose hypertension is being effectively managed on a drug regimen before they conceive often do best. With patients who present in the first trimester with hypertension that does not settle completely and permanently with rest and sedation, it has been my practice for years to initiate therapy with a small dose of a hypotensive agent such as methyldopa at that stage. The drug is continued through the mid-trimester drop and when the blood-pressure rises at about 30 weeks control can usually be obtained on an outpatient basis by increasing the dose, though hospital admission for rest and assessment may be desirable. The results of management in this way have been very satisfactory.

Hypotensive drugs have very little place in the management of pre-eclampsia, except to deal with the acute situation temporarily in fulminating pre-eclampsia. Past 32 weeks, if the lecithin-sphingomyelin ratio indicates pulmonary viability, the appropriate management of severe pre-eclampsia which does not respond to rest and sedation is to deliver the baby.

ANTIHYPERTENSIVE AGENTS
Rest and sedation

The most effective antihypertensive measure in pregnancy is rest. In mild cases of hypertension, rest at home, with careful instructions as to exactly when and how the patient should rest, and due attention to her domestic circumstances, can be of value. Hospital rest means either that the patient is in bed for 20 hours out of each 24 or is merely permitted up for toilet purposes. There is no doubt that these manoeuvres contribute heavily to reduction of both maternal risk and perinatal mortality in the hypertensive pregnancy.

The mechanism is presumably conservation of a greater proportion of the cardiac output for the uterine circulation. Morris *et al.* (1956) showed that exercise reduced myometrial blood flow markedly in pre-eclamptic patients. It seems likely from the beneficial effects on intrauterine growth that rest also improves the maternal placental circulation.

Sedatives have no direct antihypertensive effect and no direct action on the uterine circulation—they are merely an adjunct to rest. Neither barbiturates nor diazepam have been demonstrated to have adverse effects on the fetus, unless used in large doses shortly before the confinement, when a sedative withdrawal syndrome may result in the newborn. (Desmond *et al.*, 1972; Cree *et al.*, 1973).

Ganglion blockers

These drugs are mainly of historical interest in the present context. They are difficult to control, and pass the placenta, rendering the baby at risk for neonatal death from paralytic ileus if it survives delivery (Morris, 1953). There is no evidence that they improve uterine blood flow.

Protoveratrine

It is difficult to stabilize blood-pressure in the hypertensive pregnant woman with protoveratrine, which produces its hypotensive effect by the Bezold–Jarisch reflex, stimulating chemoreceptors in the heart and causing peripheral vasodilatation and cardiac deceleration via the vasomotor centre. Even if the drug is used by continuous intravenous infusion, erratic changes of blood-pressure can occur after a day or two. Though Morris (1955) found that protoveratrine improved myometrial blood flow on a short-term basis, this was not confirmed by Dixon *et al.* (1963), and fetal prognosis is not improved by either short-term use in an acute situation (Stern and Burnett, 1954) or by continued use in the third trimester (Carey, 1959). It seems unlikely that the drug has any beneficial effect on maternal placental circulation.

Reserpine

Mr J. D. Murdoch used to use small doses of this drug throughout pregnancy in mild hypertensives; the late Professor Lord Rosenheim managed some severe essential hypertensives successfully through pregnancy with the aid of a combination of a small dose of reserpine and hydrallazine. Dixon *et al.* (1963) observed that reserpine did not improve myometrial blood flow in mild essential hypertensives but this may have been because they were in late pregnancy at the time. Reserpine has gone out of favour because of its cumulative effect in depleting maternal catecholamines, the need to increase the dose to dangerous levels to cope with increasing severity of hypertension (see Hawkins, 1961), depression in the mother, and the production of a depressed baby with nasal congestion.

Hydrallazine

This drug has been shown to improve myometrial blood flow in severe pre-eclampsia (Johnson and Clayton, 1957) but it is not known if there is a corresponding improvement in maternal placental flow. It is a useful drug for controlling severe hypertension for a week or two—after that side-effects such as headaches and skin rashes tend to occur. Used with care by the intra-muscular or intravenous route in an acute exacerbation of hypertension, so as not to reduce the blood-pressure below its previous level, it does not appear to affect the fetus adversely.

Guanethidine

This is a useful drug in pregnancy, which gives stable control of blood-pressure, though there is no direct evidence of an action on uterine blood flow. An interesting feature is the rarity with which it causes postural hypo-tension in pregnancy, a common side-effect in the non-pregnant patient. It does tend to deplete catecholamines but not to a degree which would cause concern to an experienced anaesthetist aware of its use.

Methyldopa

This drug has been demonstrated to improve fetal prognosis in essential hypertension in pregnancy in controlled trials (Leather et al., 1968; Redman et al., 1976). The results of these trials confirm experience that methyldopa is not difficult to handle in pregnancy and is safe for mother and baby. Postural hypotension with methyldopa is rare in pregnancy—whether or not this is caused by the compensating effect of supine hypertension due to vena cava compression by the pregnant uterus is not clear. Fluctuations in blood-pressure are somewhat greater during a 24-hour period than with guanethi-dine but on the whole control is fairly good. The patient who is stabilized on methyldopa is no problem to an experienced anaesthetist, though the patient who has only just been started on treatment can present difficulties. The mother and sometimes the baby as well can develop a positive direct Coombs test; the mechanism of this is somewhat obscure, but it seems to have little clinical significance. Only if the maternal dose exceeds 2 g a day has meconium ileus in the baby been reported (Clark et al., 1972). If doses of methyldopa greater than 2 g a day are necessary to control hypertension, it may be desirable to reduce the dose and introduce propranolol into the regimen, even though the latter drug has its disadvantages from the point of view of the fetus.

On the other hand there is no direct evidence that methyldopa improves uterine blood flow. Leather *et al.* (1968) found that patients treated with methyldopa produced heavier babies but the average duration of gestation was longer than in their control group. Redman *et al.* (1976) were unable to show any increase in birthweight by multivariate analysis of their data, taking differences in gestational age into account.

Diuretics

Though it has been claimed that administration of chlorthiazide in pregnancy has a prophylactic effect against the development of toxaemia and reduces perinatal mortality (Finnerty and Bepko, 1966), the groups of patients studied were not strictly comparable. On the other hand the claim that, used in mild hypertension in pregnancy, the drug masks the signs of toxaemia or that it impairs fetal prognosis by causing reduction in intravascular volume are probably equally ill-founded, Menzies (1964) found no overall reduction of fetal survival though he did encounter one case of neonatal thrombocytopenic purpura, a rare side-effect. If chlorthiazide is used in doses of 1 g a day without potassium supplements, it may reduce plasma potassium levels, but this does not appear to have any clinical or electrocardiographic ill-effects in pregnancy and is in any event difficult to alter with oral potassium supplements. Chlorthiazide was first studied as an antiadrenaline agent and any beneficial effects it has in pregnancy may well be due to the mild hypotensive effect which it exhibits in a few women.

Frusemide is a much more potent diuretic and should be used with very considerable caution, if at all, in the management of hypertension in pregnancy. Liley (1970) has shown that severe hypertension in pregnancy is associated with haemoconcentration, and the additional reduction of intravascular volume which frusemide can cause may be sufficient to reduce placental perfusion. In severe cases we found it necessary to give intravenous 10% dextrose infusions to combat this effect of frusemide (Clark *et al.*, 1972).

Diazoxide

Obstetricians are reluctant to employ a possibly diabetogenic drug in the potentially diabetogenic state of pregnancy, and diazoxide has not been used much in hypertensive pregnancies. It can also cause hyperuricaemia. The dramatic and persisting fall in blood-pressure that a bolus injection can produce is known to reduce renal blood flow (Johnson, 1971) and may easily impair perfusion of sclerotic placental blood-vessels and endanger the fetus. On continued administration in hypertensives diazoxide is known to improve perfusion of the renal circulation (Hamby *et al.*, 1968) but it is not clear that it has any comparable effect on the uterine circulation. In pregnant baboons slow intravenous infusions of the drug do not affect the fetuses adversely (Morishima *et al.*, 1976).

28

Propranolol

This beta-sympatholytic agent would be expected to prevent adrenergic dilatation in the uterine circulation—in sheep it has been shown to antagonize the vasodilator effect of isoprenaline on the myometrial blood flow (Greiss, 1972). This may cause little harm in the patient whose placental reserve is good, but to reduce blood-pressure in a hypertensive patient with a drug that prevents placental vasodilatation may place the fetus in jeopardy. Propranolol in pregnancy should be reserved for (a) patients with cardiomyopathy or paroxysmal tachycardia, where it is indicated on cardiac grounds, (b) patients presenting in pregnancy on a stable regimen including propranolol, established before the pregnancy, which the physician is reluctant to disturb, (c) patients whose blood-pressure is rising out of control on reasonable doses of methyldopa, where incorporation of propranolol into the regimen enables control.

Beta-sympathomimetics

There is fairly good evidence that the beta receptors in the utero-placental circulation mediate vasodilatation. What is not established is that the maternal vessels supplying the placenta are dilated or that perfusion of the placenta is improved by administration of beta-sympathomimetics. In fact, Greiss (1972) has shown in the sheep that whilst isoprenaline increases myometrial blood flow by a mechanism which is antagonized by propranolol, in the presence of the intact placental circulation increased blood flow in response to a beta-sympathomimetic could not be demonstrated. This suggests that the response of the myometrial vessels may actually impair the flow through the maternal placenta.

In the pregnant woman there is evidence, obtained with thermistor probes that the intravenous infusion of isoxsuprine increases flow through the uterine artery (Brotánek and Hodr, 1967). Somewhat disconcerting was the observation of excessive fetal movements—a traditional sign of fetal distress—when the infusion was discontinued. Brettes et al. (1976) has shown in placebo controlled studies with thermistors that ritodrine infusions increase uterine blood flow, but only in hypertensive pregnant patients. Similar results have been obtained using placental clearance of radioactive technesium or indium—improved blood flow in hypertensive pregnancy but no effect if the blood-pressure is normal (Janisch et al., 1972; Renaud et al., 1976). In contrast Suonio et al. (1975) could only show that isoxsuprine increased uterine blood flow in normal pregnancies, perhaps the uterine vessels of their hypertensive patients were too sclerotic to respond. The effects of infusions of ritodrine (Gamissans et al., 1972; Renaud et al., 1972) or orciprenaline (Angiolillo, 1972) in relieving fetal distress in labour is consistent with the view that beta-sympathomimetics improve maternal placental blood flow.

It has been thought that ritodrine administered chronically might have a beneficial effect on intrauterine growth of the fetus, presumably by improving uterine blood flow, but Seidl *et al.* (1972) were unable to confirm this. We have used oral isoxsuprine as part of a drug regimen in severe hypertension in pregnancy (Clark *et al.*, 1972), but complexity of the variables prohibited assessment. We did establish that if full oral doses of isoxsuprine (20 mg or more) are given they must be administered after meals to delay absorption, and the patient should preferably be confined to bed, if hypotensive responses sufficient to cause syncope and fetal distress are to be avoided. Dose of beta-sympathomimetics is also limited by maternal tachycardia and side-effects such as anxiety.

Clonidine

There is as yet no information on the effects of clonidine on the uterine blood flow. Obstetricians are justifiably conservative about the use of drugs in pregnancy, and clonidine is perhaps best avoided until considerably more is known about its mode of action and complex side-effects. The tendency of the drug to cause an initial elevation of blood-pressure would suggest that its use should at least be confined to patients whose blood-pressure is well controlled on a regimen including clonidine before they become pregnant.

Epidural anaesthesia

This is only of use in controlling blood-pressure during labour or possibly for a short period during an acute exacerbation. Findings with epidural block are of some interest in that they illustrate the general principles of the use of antihypertensive measures. Brotánek *et al.* (1973) have shown with a thermistor probe that epidural block had no effect on uterine blood flow unless systemic hypotension occurred, when the flow was reduced. Pre-eclamptic patients were particularly prone to this effect. Clinical observations are entirely compatible with this. The patient should be kept in the left lateral position as far as possible to avoid supine hypotension. If blood-pressure of hypertensive patients is controlled by the epidural block during labour to a level comparable to that existing before, then no harm to the baby results (James and Davies, 1976). If maternal hypotension occurs, then fetal distress and acidosis result, probably due to the reduced perfusion pressure and uterine blood flow. Greiss (1967) feels that if maternal hypotension occurs with an epidural block it should be treated by rapid fluid infusion rather than by alpha-sympathomimetics. This seems logical as it should increase tissue perfusion, whilst the alpha receptor stimulants could cause vasoconstriction in the utero-placental circulation. On the other hand,

Shnider *et al.* (1968) never found that ephedrine used to counteract spinal hypotension endangered the fetus.

FULMINATING PRE-ECLAMPSIA AND ECLAMPSIA

In the past 25 years no single procedure has been evolved which has been proved to really reduce the high perinatal mortality of these conditions except for the prompt use of Caesarean section under general anaesthesia (Kyank *et al.*, 1964). Nonetheless, the principles of preservation of uterine blood flow should be borne in mind in selecting an approach which gives the fetus the best chance of survival from amongst those which will preserve the mother. Of the drugs now available only protoveratrine (Morris, 1953), hydrallazine (Johnson and Clayton, 1957) and chlorpromazine (Cliff *et al.*, 1963) have been found to dilate at least the myometrial vessels. Careful use of procedures employing one of these drugs with avoidance of abrupt fall in blood-pressure which can result in intrauterine death of the fetus, may give the best chance of a live baby.

CONCLUSION

The demonstration by Carey (1959) that protoveratrine used in the third trimester would protect the hypertensive mother but not improve fetal prognosis had a profound inhibitory effect on the therapeutics of hypertension in pregnancy. It was left to those with faith in the principle that control of blood-pressure throughout pregnancy tends to preserve uterine blood flow and result in a live baby to pursue the use of hypotensive drugs. The demonstrations by Leather *et al.* (1968) and Redman *et al.* (1976) that use of methyldopa can improve fetal prognosis should be an encouragement to investigators to study the role of uterine blood flow responses in more depth, although the methodology is so difficult.

References

Angiolillo, M. (1972). Medical treatment of acute foetal distress. In K. Baumgarten and A. Wessalius-de Casparis (eds.) *Proceedings of the International Symposium on the Treatment of Foetal Risks*, pp. 152–156. (University of Vienna)

Bienarz, J., Yoshida, T., Romero-Salinas, G., Curuchet, E., Caldeyro-Barcia, R. and Crottogini, J. J. (1969). Aortocaval compression by the uterus in late human pregnancy; IV. Circulatory homeostasis by preferential perfusion of the placenta. *Am. J. Obstet. Gynecol.*, **103**, 19

Blechner, J. N., Stenger, V. G. and Prystowsky, H. (1974). Uterine blood flow in women at term. *Am. J. Obstet. Gynecol.*, **120**, 633

Brettes, J. P., Renaud, R. and Gandar, R. (1976). A double-blind investigation into the effects of ritodrine on uterine blood flow during the third trimester of pregnancy. *Am. J. Obstet. Gynecol.*, **124**, 164

Brotánek, V. and Hodr, J. (1967). The effect of isoxsuprine on utero-placental circulation. In J. Horský and Z. K. Štembera (eds.) *Intra-Uterine Dangers to the Foetus*, pp. 424–427. (Amsterdam: Excerpta Medica)

Brotánek, V., Vasicka, A., Santiago, A. and Brotánek, J. D. A. (1973). The influence of epidural anaesthesia on uterine blood flow. *Obstet. Gynecol., N.Y.*, **42**, 276

Browne, J. C. M. and Veall, N. (1953). The maternal placental blood flow in normotensive and hypertensive women. *J. Obstet. Gynaecol. Br. Commonw.*, **60**, 141

Bruce, N. W. and Abdul-Karim, R. W. (1974). Mechanisms controlling maternal placental circulation. *Clin. Obstet. Gynecol.*, **17**, 135

Carey, H. M. (1959). Protoveratrine in the treatment of hypertension during pregnancy. *N. Z. Med. J.*, **58**, 467

Clark, A. D., Sevitt, L. H. and Hawkins, D. F. (1972). Use of frusemide in severe toxaemia of pregnancy. *Lancet*, **i**, 35

Cliff, W. J., Martin, J. D. and Michael, C. A. (1963). Use of ear chamber with uterine muscle transplant to differentiate myometrial and vascular activity. *Nature (London)*, **199**, 399

Cox, L. W., Munday, R. N. and Sauer, H. H. A. (1963). The use of radioactive isotopes in determining placental function. *Aust. N. Z. J. Obstet. Gynaecol.*, **3**, 119

Cree, J. E., Meyer, J. and Harley, D. M. (1973). Diazepam in labour: metabolism and effect on clinical condition and thermogenesis of newborn. *Br. Med. J.*, **4**, 251

Desmond, M. M., Schwanecke, R. P., Wilson, G. S., Yasugaga, S. and Burgdorff, I. (1972). Maternal barbiturate utilization and neonatal withdrawal symptomatology. *J. Pediatr.*, **80**, 190

Dixon, H. G., Browne, J. C. M. and Davey, D. A. (1963). Choriodecidual and myometrial blood-flow. *Lancet*, **ii**, 369

Finnerty, F. A. and Bepko, F. J. (1966). Lowering the perinatal mortality and the prematurity rate. The value of prophylactic thiazides in juveniles. *J. Am. Med. Assoc.*, **195**, 429

Gamissans, O., Carreras, M., Durán, P., Cararach, J., Calaf, J., Abril, V. and Esteban-Altirriba, J. (1972). The treatment of fetal acidosis with beta-mimetic drugs. Studies on acid–base balance, blood glucose levels and uterine motility. In K. Baumgarten and A. Wessalius-de Casparis (eds.) *Proceedings of the International Symposium on the Treatment of Foetal Risks*, pp. 145–148. (University of Vienna)

Greiss, F. C., Jr. (1967). A clinical concept of uterine blood flow during pregnancy. *Obstet. Gynecol., N.Y.*, **30**, 595

Greiss, F. C., Jr. (1972). Differential reactivity of the myoendometrial and placental vasculatures: adrenergic responses. *Am. J. Obstet. Gynecol.*, **112**, 20

Greiss, F. C., Jr. (1974). Uterine blood flow in women at term. Discussion. *Am. J. Obstet. Gynecol.*, **120**, 638

Hamby, W. M., Jankowski, G. J., Pouget, J. M., Dunea, G. and Gantt, C. L. (1968). Intravenous use of diazoxide in the treatment of severe hypertension. *Circulation*, **37**, 169

Hawkins, D. F. (1961). Collapse from reserpine. *Br. Med. J.*, **1**, 1465

Jacoby, H. E., Arnot, R. N., Glass, H. I. and Browne, J. C. M. (1972). Estimation of clearance rate of inhaled xenon-133 in the placental region of the pregnant uterus. *J. Obstet. Gynaecol. Br. Commonw.*, **79**, 531

James, F. M., III, and Davies, P. (1976). Maternal and fetal effects of lumbar epidural anasthesia for labor and delivery in patients with gestational hypertension. *Am. J. Obstet. Gynecol.*, **126**, 195

Janisch, H., Leodolter, S. and Reinold, E. (1972). Der effekt von ritodrine auf die plazentadurchblutung. In K. Baumgarten and A. Wessalius-de Casparis (eds.) *Proceedings of the International Symposium on the Treatment of Foetal Risks*, pp. 51–52. (University of Vienna)

Johnson, B. F. (1971). Diazoxide and renal function in man. *Clin. Pharmac. Ther.*, **12**, 815

Johnson, T. and Clayton, C. G. (1957). Diffusion of radioactive sodium in normotensive and pre-eclamptic pregnancies. *Br. Med. J.*, **1**, 312

ANTIHYPERTENSIVE DRUGS AND UTERINE BLOOD FLOW

Kyank, H., Schubert, E. and Gyöngyössy, A. (1964). Evaluation of cases of eclampsia treated between 1957 and 1960 at 72 German obstetric clinics: comparison with a similar series treated between 1959 and 1961 at 97 Hungarian clinics. *Germ. Med. Mon.*, **9**, 108

Leather, H. M., Humphreys, D. M., Baker, P. and Chadd, M. A. (1968). A controlled trial of hypotensive agents in hypertension in pregnancy. *Lancet*, **ii**, 488

Liley, A. W. (1970). Clinical and laboratory significance of variations in maternal plasma volume in pregnancy. *J. Int. Fed. Gynecol. Obstet.*, **8**, 358

Menzies, D. N. (1964). Controlled trial of chlorthiazide in treatment of early pre-eclampsia. *Br Med. J.*, **1**, 739

Morishima, H. O., Caritis, S. N., Yeh, M. N. and James, L. S. (1976). Prolonged infusion of diazoxide in the management of premature labor in the baboon. *Obstet. Gynecol., N.Y.*, **48**, 203

Morris, N. (1953). Hexamethonium compounds in the treatment of pre-eclampsia and essential hypertension in pregnancy. *Proc. R. Soc. Med.*, **46**, 402

Morris, N. (1955). The treatment of imminent eclampsia. *J. Obstet. Gynaecol. Br. Commonw.*, **62**, 696

Morris, N., Osborn, S. B. and Wright, H. P. (1955). Effective circulation of the uterine wall in late pregnancy. *Lancet*, **i**, 323

Morris, N., Osborn, S. B., Wright, H. P. and Hart, A. (1956). Effective uterine blood flow during exercise in normal and pre-eclamptic pregnancies. *Lancet*, **ii**, 481

Prill, H. J. and Götz, F. (1961). Blood flow in the myometrium and endometrium of the uterus. *Am. J. Obstet. Gynecol.*, **82**, 102

Redman, C. W. G., Beilin, L. J., Bonnar, J. and Oansted, M. K. (1976). Fetal outcome in trial of antihypertensive treatment in pregnancy. *Lancet*, **ii**, 753

Renaud, R., Bock, A., Chanbron, J., Bonnafous, J., Rosenthal, C. and Raffi, F. (1976). Étude simultanée des circulations placentaire, myometriale et cervicale (indium-133 et thermometric anenometrique). *J. Gynecol. Obstet. Biol. Reprod.*, **5**, 611

Renaud, R., Brettes, P., Boog, G., Irrmann, M., Schumacher, J. C., van Lierde, M. and Gandar, R. (1972). The place of beta-mimetics in the treatment of acute foetal distress during labour. In K. Baumgarten and A. Wessalius-de Casparis (eds.) *Proceedings of the International Symposium on the Treatment of Foetal Risks*, pp. 177–179. (University of Vienna)

Robertson, W. B., Brosens, I. and Dixon, H. G. (1967). The pathological response of the vessels of the placental bed to hypertensive pregnancy. *J. Pathol. Bacteriol.*, **93**, 581

Seidl, A., Baumgarten, K., Eisner, R., Fröheich, H., Gruber, W. and Urban, G. (1972). Auswirkung der ritodrinebehandlung auf das kindesgewicht. (1972). In K. Baumgarten and A. Wessalius-de Casparis (eds.) *Proceedings of the International Symposium on the Treatment of Foetal Risks*, pp. 61–63. (University of Vienna)

Shnider, S. M., De Lorimer, A. A., Holl, J. W., Chapler, F. K. and Morishima, H. O. (1968). Vasopressors in obstetrics I. Correction of fetal acidosis with ephedrine during spinal hypotension. *Am. J. Obstet. Gynecol.*, **102**, 911

Stern, D. M. and Burnett, C. W. F. (1954). An evaluation of modern treatment of eclampsia. *J. Obstet. Gynaecol. Br. Emp.*, **61**, 590

Suonio, S., Jalkanen, M., Olkkonen, H. and Castrén, O. (1975). Effect of isoxsuprine on uteroplacental blood flow in normal and hypertensive patients during the last trimester of pregnancy. *J. Int. Fed. Gynecol. Obstet.*, **13**, 225

Theobald, G. W. (1961). The importance of placentation evidenced by denervation of the internal iliac vessels. *J. Obstet. Gynaecol. Br. Commonw.*, **68**, 197

Wigglesworth, J. S. (1964). Experimental growth retardation in the fetal rat. *J. Pathol. Bacteriol.*, **88**, 1

3
The Effect
of Antihypertensive
Drugs on the Fetus

G. S. DAWES

FETAL PHARMACOLOGY

Until the thalidomide disaster there had been relatively little interest in the effect of drugs on the embryo or fetus. Before this most drug studies had been carried out on adult animals. Thalidomide changed all this, and it is now mandatory for new drugs to be screened for their effects in pregnancy. However, the effects sought are morphological changes in the embryo; there has been little interest in the more subtle effect of drugs later in pregnancy, when morphogenesis is largely complete and the fetus is growing rapidly. Indeed, in clinical obstetrics there is much the same casual attitude towards the use of new drugs in the last trimester of pregnancy as once there was towards the use of new drugs in the first trimester. Systematic animal fetal pharmacology is not carried out on new drugs; the sum of knowledge on the effect of drugs on the fetus is small. There are some signs that interest in this field is beginning. Symposia are being held (e.g. Boreus, 1973) and incidental observations on fetal pharmacology made during the course of physiological experiments are now beginning to be collated.

ANTIHYPERTENSIVE DRUGS AND THE FETUS

The present unsatisfactory situation in fetal pharmacology is well illustrated by our knowledge of the effect of antihypertensive agents on the fetus. The use of antihypertensive drugs in the general population is increasing. There are several reasons for this. There is greater awareness amongst physicians of the long-term hazards of raised arterial pressure, so that patients with mild and asymptomatic hypertension are now being actively treated with drugs. This trend is facilitated by the availability of acceptable antihypertensive drugs with few side effects. Inevitably among the women taking these drugs some will become pregnant. Furthermore obstetricians now consider treating women with raised arterial pressure first discovered during pregnancy. Yet the fetal effects of these drugs have been little investigated in animals. A particular example is that of the beta-blockers.

FETAL EFFECTS OF BETA-ADRENOCEPTOR ANTAGONISTS

Beta-blockers are now widely used for the treatment of hypertension. Their use has increased since the first discovery that propranolol was an effective antihypertensive agent with few side-effects. Incidentally the way in which these drugs lower blood-pressure is still unknown. Almost 10 years ago I was consulted about the likely consequences which would result if the human fetus was exposed to propranolol being taken by its mother. It was known that propranolol crossed the mammalian placenta (Masuoka and Hanssen, 1967). On theoretical grounds I was concerned that such exposure might have a serious consequence for the fetus for the following reasons.

Thermogenesis

First, as Hull (1964) has shown, non-shivering thermogenesis in the newborn mammal is dependent on beta-adrenergic stimulation of brown adipose tissue and this process is inhibited by beta-blockade. Since human babies also depend on this mechanism for thermal control in the immediate postnatal period it was likely that babies born to mothers who had been given propranolol up until delivery might be less able to control their body temperatures and would thus be at greater risk from hypothermia.

Cardiac effects

More importantly, it was likely that the blockade by propranolol of the positive chronotropic effects of catecholamines on the fetal heart which had, not surprisingly, already been observed in the lamb by 1968 (unpublished observations) would at least obtund the heart-rate changes on which obstetricians depended to assess fetal health. This in itself might be hazardous, leading to unnecessary interventions in the pregnancy or conversely lack of awareness that a fetus was at risk. Quite apart from these diagnostic considerations the effects of beta-blockers in abolishing the inotropic effects of catecholamines (i.e. the increase in the contractility of the fetal heart) should limit the ability of the fetus to maintain its internal environment, especially in hypoxia.

Metabolic effects

Finally, since it was known that catecholamines exert metabolic effects in adults, then in the fetus blockade of these effects might also be harmful. In view of these considerations it seemed prudent to suggest that if beta-blockers were to be widely used then a programme of animal experiments would be desirable to define what the effect of the drug was likely to be on the human fetus. At least this would allow a warning to be issued about the possible consequences of fetal beta-blockade.

At present it appears that very little *systematic* investigation has been done and furthermore many of these theoretical predictions have had some unfortunate counterparts in clinical practice, such as neonatal hypoglycaemia (Fiddler, 1974; Gladstone *et al.*, 1975) and bradycardia (Reed *et al.*, 1974). Ironically most of the published work on propranolol in pregnancy relates to the clinical experience of obstetricians managing women taking the drug for cardiac disease (Goodwin and Oakley, 1972) or thyrotoxicosis (Langer *et al.*, 1974). And it is astonishing to relate that in some of these clinical investigations no systematic study was undertaken even of the fetal heart rate. Deliberate animal experimentation on the effect of beta-blockade on the fetus has lagged behind. Clearly this is a most undesirable situation.

BETA-BLOCKADE IN THE ANIMAL FETUS

Such animal work which has been done has not been reassuring. van Petter and Willes (1970; 1973) reported that the unanaesthetized sheep fetus responded to isoprenaline given intravenously with tachycardia; this was antagonized by propranolol given to the mother. It was noted that the blockade of the isoprenaline response in the fetus persisted much longer than in the mother and this delayed effect might be potentially harmful. In 1973 the same group (Truelove *et al.*, 1973) investigated the effects on the sheep fetus of several different beta-adrenoceptor blocking agents. Oxprenolol, propranolol and bunolol produced fetal beta-blockade when given to the mother. Sotalol and several other beta-blockers not used clinically did not cause blockade in the fetus when given to pregnant ewes. Of the beta-blockers tested which produced fetal beta-blockade propranolol and oxprenolol produced prolonged blockade in the fetus. There was a good correlation between the lipid solubility of the drug and the degree of beta-blockade suggesting that the important difference between the beta-blockers which affected the fetus and those which did not was their ability to traverse the ovine placenta. This work suggested that the more lipophobic beta-blockers such as sotalol, practolol, metroprolol and atenolol, might produce less beta-blockade in the human fetus. On theoretical grounds these beta-blockers might be preferred during pregnancy to the more lipid soluble beta-blockers. As far as I am aware sotalol, metoprolol and atenolol have not been studied in human pregnancy. There are some studies with practolol (McDevitt *et al.*, 1975) in women, suggesting that it does not produce fetal beta-blockade. However, practolol has been withdrawn from clinical use for other reasons.

Drs C. T. Jones and J. W. K. Ritchie (personal communication) have studied the effect of propranolol on the metabolic responses to intravenous infusion of catecholamines in the fetal lamb. Propranolol administered to the mother had three effects. It decreased the rise in plasma glucose and lactate normally induced in the fetus by catecholamine infusion. Propranolol also abolished the rise in plasma-free fatty acids in the fetus and the rise in plasma amino nitrogen. All three specific metabolic effects of catecholamines, mobilization of carbohydrate, lipid and amino acids were reduced or blocked by beta-blockade. During fetal hypoxia there is a release of catecholamines (Jones and Robinson, 1975) and a rise in fetal plasma glucose, lactate and free fatty acids; it would seem unwise to block these metabolic responses without much further information.

BETA-BLOCKERS, THE HEART AND FETAL HYPOXIA

J. Milligan and J. F. Goodwin (personal communication) measured fetal dp/dt as an index of myocardial contractility in the lamb and observed that in acute hypoxia fetal left ventricular contractility rose (when studied in the last third of gestation). This is consistent with the large rise in plasma catecholamines, as high as $10 \, \mu g/l$, observed by Jones and Robinson (1975). These observations suggest that the release of catecholamines is an important fetal response to hypoxia. One consequence of this catecholamine release is an increase in left ventricular contractility and hence maintenance of cardiac output against a rise in peripheral resistance. The cardiac effects of catecholamines are of course antagonized by beta-blockade (e.g. Joelsson *et al.*, 1972).

Other more recent work on hypoxia in the sheep fetus has confirmed the original theoretical hypothesis that beta-blockade would impair the circulatory response to hypoxia. With prolonged hypoxia there is a fall in cardiac output although umbilical blood flow is preferentially preserved. The explanation for the latter is that between 40 and 45% of the combined output of both left and right ventricles goes to the placenta in the lamb and this umbilical circulation is very insensitive to vasoactive agents. However, the fetal body tissues are relatively sensitive to vasoactive drugs and during hypoxia catecholamines constrict resistance vessels in the muscle and skin of the fetus allowing an increased proportion of the diminished cardiac output to reach the umbilical circulation. In the presence of propranolol not only is total cardiac output further diminished but the proportion that goes to the fetal side of the placenta also is diminished (Cohn *et al.*, 1977). The hypoxic fetus is therefore further compromised by the presence of beta-blockers. As long ago as 1972 Hyman *et al.* showed the danger of combined alpha- and beta-blockade in fetal hypoxia There have been several unpublished observations among those who work with fetal lambs, of the dangers of beta-blockade alone.

DEVELOPMENT OF CIRCULATORY CONTROL IN THE MAMMALIAN FETUS

These considerations apply to the fetus in the last third of gestation. In the first two-thirds of gestation, control of the circulation is not dependent upon the autonomic nervous system nor the renin angiotensin system to a very important degree. These systems assume control in the last third of pregnancy. Some experiments which illustrate the change in the way in which the fetal circulation is regulated with maturity of the pregnancy are shown in

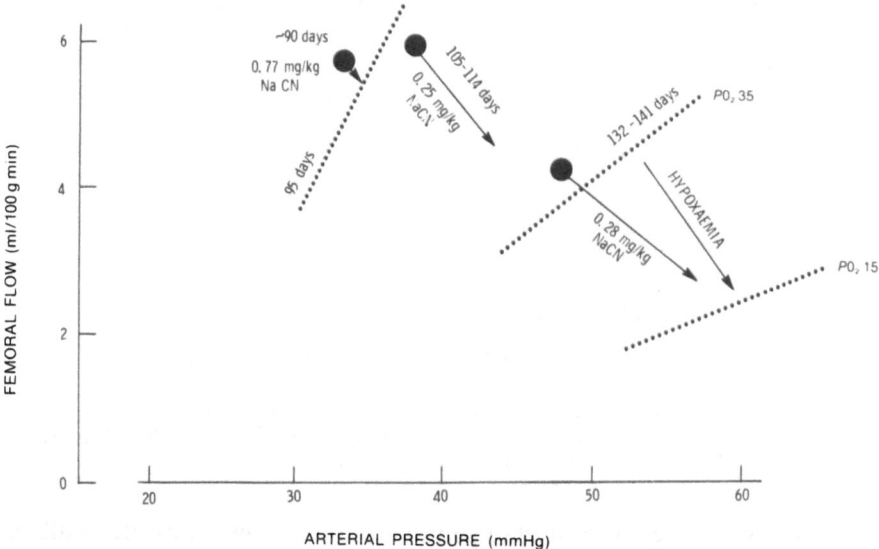

Figure 3.1 The effect of injecting NaCN in fetal lambs. With increasing gestational age the vasoconstriction in the hind limbs (as shown by the shift in the pressure–flow relationship) becomes greater (modified from Dawes *et al.*, 1968)

Figure 3.1. This shows the result of injecting cyanide in the fetal lamb. At 95 days, two-thirds of the way through ovine gestation, the effect of cyanide is negligible. At about 110 days there is a small hind limb vasoconstrictor response to cyanide and during the last sixth of gestation the cyanide causes very severe vasoconstriction. The vasoconstriction can be blocked with alpha-adrenoceptor blocking drugs. These observations illustrate rather

39

neatly the developing importance of the peripheral sympathetic nervous system as the fetus matures.

Another illustration of this kind of change is shown in Figure 3.2 in which very small doses of pentobarbitone were given to pregnant ewes. There was no effect on the mother. However, interesting effects were observed on the fetus, varying with age. Again observations were made on fetuses at 90 days, 120 days and near term (147 days). With increased fetal age the basal fetal

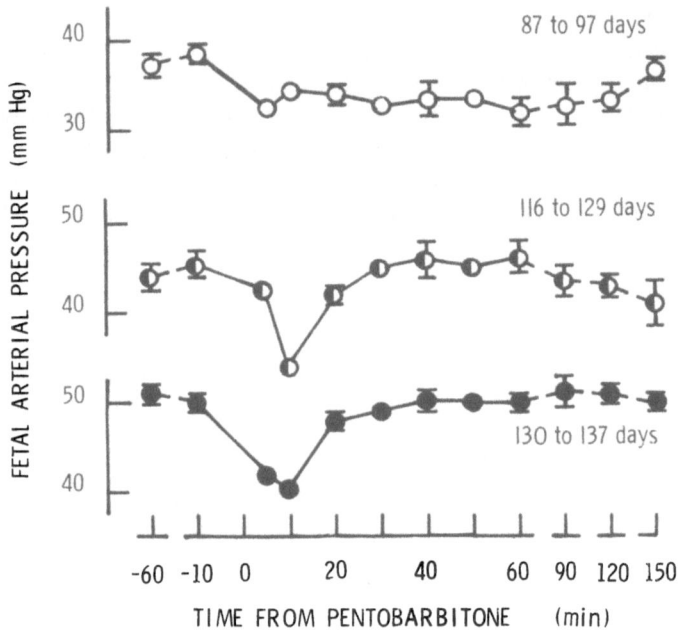

Figure 3.2 The effect of pentobarbitone (4 mg/kg given to the ewe) on arterial pressure in the fetal lamb at different periods of gestation (reprinted from Boddy *et al.* (1976) *Br. J. Pharmacol.*, **57**, 311, by kind permission of the authors and publishers)

blood-pressure rises. The effect of pentobarbitone is comparatively small on the fetuses of 90 days which have very little vasoconstrictor tone. With increasing age the small dose of pentobarbitone (4 mg/kg i.v. to the ewe over 2 min) caused larger falls in arterial pressure. The pentobarbitone presumably depresses the central nervous mechanisms which regulate the autonomic nervous system. These assume greater importance as the pregnancy proceeds.

A similar increasing effect of pentobarbitone is seen when the heart-rate responses of the fetuses are studied (Figure 3.3). The fetal heart-rate falls progressively through pregnancy and this is believed to be due to a progressive increase in vagal tone and also a decrease in innate pacemaker rate as the fetus matures (Walker, 1974). In the near-term fetus where the autonomic nervous system has taken a predominant role in the regulation of heart-rate, the hypotensive effect of pentobarbitone induces a compensatory tachycardia. These results demonstrate that the effects of administering drugs to the mother would depend on the gestational age of the fetus. The effect of propranolol on fetal heart-rate in the lamb is greater towards term (Vapaavouri *et al.*, 1973). All the indications are therefore that in the human fetus between 28 weeks and term the circulation has become largely regulated by the autonomic nervous system and thus susceptible to interference by autonomic blocking drugs given to the mother.

In summary these considerations make it likely that propranolol and other beta-blockers which gain access to the fetus will interfere with the regulation of the fetal circulation. These effects will be particularly great in the fetus which becomes hypoxic. Some of the effects of hypoxia will be masked and the metabolic and cardiovascular responses to hypoxia will be blocked.

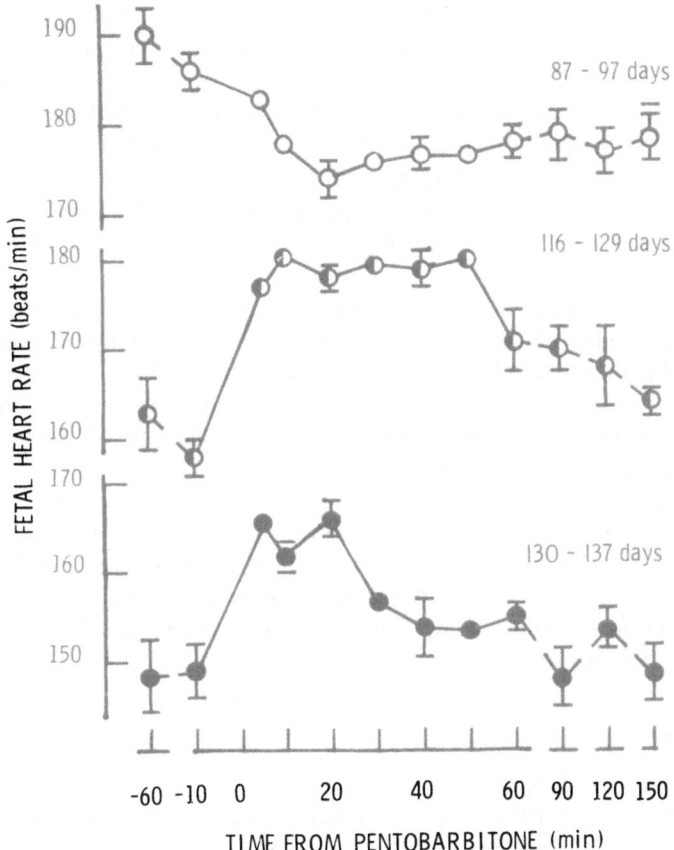

Figure 3.3 The effect of pentobarbitone (as in Figure 3.2) on heart rate in the fetal lamb at different periods of gestation (reprinted from Boddy *et al.* (1976) *Br. J. Pharmacol.*, **57**, 311, by kind permission of the authors and publishers)

Once it was realized that propranolol would gain access to the fetus then all these effects were predictable, and although there is not enough clinical data to document adverse effects in a completely convincing way, not enough work has been done to show that these effects can be ignored.

EFFECTS OF OTHER DRUGS ON THE FETUS

This situation which I have described with beta-blocking drugs is not unique. In recent years several interesting developments have occurred in obstetric therapeutics. More drugs are being used to treat the pregnant woman near term. A good example is the use of betamethasone to increase the production of pulmonary surfactant in the premature fetus. The effect on the fetus of betamethasone administration to the mother has not been systematically investigated in animals and there is one disturbing observation. Ryan and Challis (1976) demonstrated in rhesus monkeys that dexamethasone administered to the mother suppressed the production of steroids by the fetal adrenal cortex, and caused atrophy of the fetal zone. We do not know the consequences to premature neonates of their being delivered with impaired corticosteroid production. Obviously the beneficial effects of inducing surfactant have to be balanced against other effects. But this observation on adrenal suppression is not widely appreciated and it is disturbing that so little interest has been taken in the broader endocrine aspect of this new therapy.

Another case in point is that of the prostaglandin synthetase inhibitor indomethacin which is being used to suppress premature labour. In addition to inhibiting prostaglandin synthesis in the mother, the drug may inhibit prostaglandin synthesis in the fetus. The effects of suppressing fetal and newborn prostaglandin production have not been systematically investigated. Other examples could be cited.

It is disturbing that there seems to be little national interest in the problem of fetal pharmacology. Obstetricians today are faced with the problem of deciding whether or not to use new drug treatments and yet they have not been provided with the necessary information as to the likely effect of these drugs on the fetus. There is little indication that efforts are being made to remedy this situation.

References

Boddy, K., Dawes, G. S., Fischer, R. L., Pinter, S. and Robinson, J. S. (1976). The effects of pentobarbitone and pethidine on foetal breathing movements in sheep. *Br. J. Pharmacol.*, **57**, 311

Boreus, L. O. (1973). *Fetal Pharmacology*. (New York: Raven Press)

Challis, J. R. G., Davies, I. J., Benirschke, K., Hendrick, A. G. and Ryan, K. (1974). The effects of dexamethasone on plasma steroid levels and fetal adrenal histology in the pregnant rhesus monkey. *J. Endocrinol.*, **95**, 1300

ANTIHYPERTENSIVE DRUGS AND THE FETUS

Cohn, H. E., Piasecki, G. J. and Jackson, B. T. (1977). In L. Longo (ed.) *Circulation in the Fetus and Newborn*. (In press) (Berlin: Springer Verlag)

Dawes, G. S., Lewis, B. V., Milligan, J. E., Roach, M. R. and Talner, N. S. (1968). Vasomotor responses in the hind limbs of foetal and newborn lambs to asphyxia and aortic chemoreceptor stimulation. *J. Physiol.*, **195**, 55

Fiddler, G. I. (1974). Propranolol and pregnancy. *Lancet*, **ii**, 722

Gladstone, G. R., Hordo, F. A. and Gersony, W. M. (1975). Propranolol administration during pregnancy: effects on the fetus. *J. Paediatr.*, **86**, 962

Goodwin, J. F. and Oakley, C. M. (1972). The cardiomyopathies. *Br. Heart J.*, **34**, 545

Hull, D. (1964). Pronethalol and the oxygen consumption of newborn rabbits. *J. Physiol.*, **173**, 13

Hyman, A. I., Haworth, G., Bowe, E. T., Daniel, S. S. and James, L. S. (1972). Effects of sympathetic blockade on the fetal responses to asphyxia. *Biol. Neonate*, **21**, 1

Joelsson, I., Barton, M. D., Daniel, S., James, S. and Adamsons, K. (1972). The response of the unanesthetized sheep fetus to sympathomimetic amines and adrenergic blocking agents. *Am. J. Obstet. Gynecol.*, **114**, 43

Jones, C. T. and Ritchie, J. W. K. (1976). Endocrine and metabolic changes associated with periods of spontaneous hypoxia in fetal sheep. *Biol. Neonate*, **29**, 286

Jones, C. T. and Robinson, R. O. (1975). Plasma catecholamines in fetal and adult sheep. *J. Physiol.*, **248**, 15

Langer, A. Hung, C. T., McA'nulty, J. A., Harrigan, J. T. and Washington, E. (1974). Adrenergic blockade. A new approach to hyperthyroidism during pregnancy. *Obstet. Gynecol.*, **44**, 181

McDevitt, D. G., Wallace, R. J., Roberts, A. and Whitfield, C. R. (1975). The uterine and cardiovascular effects of salbutamol and practolol during labour. *Br. J. Obstet. Gynaecol.*, **82**, 442

Masuoka, D. and Hanssen, E. (1967). Autoradiographic distribution studies of adrenergic blocking agents. II. 14C-propranolol beta-receptor-type blocker. *Acta. Pharmacol. Toxicol.*, **25**, 447

van Petten, G. R. and Willes, R. F. (1970). Beta-adrenoceptive responses in the unanaesthetised ovine foetus. *Br. J. Pharmacol.*, **38**, 572

van Petten, G. R. (1973). Placental transfer and foetal effects of drugs which modify adrenergic function. In: *Fetal and Neonatal Physiology, Proceedings of the Sir J. Barcroft Symposium*, p. 164. (Cambridge: Cambridge University Press)

Reed, R. L., Cheney, C. B., Fearon, R. E., Hook, R. and Hehre, F. W. (1974). Propranolol therapy throughout pregnancy: a case report. *Anaesth. Analges.*, **53**, 214

Truelove, J. F., van Petten, G. R. and Willes, R. F. (1973). Action of several adrenoceptor blocking drugs in the pregnant sheep and fetus. *Br. J. Pharmacol.*, **47**, 161

Vapaavouri, E. K., Shinebourne, E. A., Williams, R. L., Heymann, M. A. and Rudolph, A. M. (1973). Development of cardiovascular responses to autonomic blockade in intact fetal and neonatal lambs. *Biol. Neonate*, **22**, 177

Walker, D. (1974). *In vitro* observations on the function of the sino-arterial node in the human fetus, without a comment on the fetal heart rate throughout pregnancy. *Biol. Neonate*, **24**, 138

Discussion

O'Grady, J., Beckenham: In view of the fact that pentobarbitone has effects on arterial pressure and heart rate in the fetal lamb, do you think that the human fetus is similarly affected when women are treated with barbiturates during pregnancy as is done for pre-eclamptic toxaemia?

Dawes: This is a very good example of the problem we face. So far as I am aware there have been no systematic studies of the effect of phenobarbitone given to the mother on the fetus. This is a commonly used drug and yet there is no information as to its circulatory effects.

Dollery: The effect of barbiturates given for pre-eclampsia have been investigated on drug metabolism in the fetus but I also know of no data on cardiovascular effects.

4
Fetal Outcome in Pregnancies Complicated by Severe Hypertension Treated with Propranolol

G. M. STIRRAT and B. A. LIEBERMAN

Despite the availability of hypotensive agents for over 20 years, there have only been two controlled trials to assess their value in pregnancy hypertension. Leather *et al.* (1968) using methyldopa and a thiazide diuretic, suggested that the prognosis was improved by treatment before 20 weeks gestation. Redman *et al.* (1976) found an improved fetal outcome in those patients treated with methyldopa from a group of 242 women with 'moderate' pregnancy hypertension allocated randomly to 'treatment' and 'no-treatment' groups. Other uncontrolled series have indicated that the use of methyldopa is safe in pregnancy (Hans and Kopelman, 1964; Kincaid-Smith *et al.*, 1966) but the value of other drugs is far from clear (Feitelson and Lindheimer, 1972).

Beta-adrenergic blockade, most frequently by propranolol, has now established itself as a valuable method for controlling hypertension outwith pregnancy (Prichard and Gillam, 1969; Holland and Kaplan, 1976). This has inevitably meant that some women have become pregnant on such treatment while others have had propranolol prescribed for the first time during pregnancy. Because of the report of Joelsson *et al.*, suggesting that beta-blockade rendered fetal lambs less capable of responding to anoxia, it was decided to review retrospectively the fetal outcome in those patients suffering from pregnancy hypertension who had been treated with propranolol and/or other hypotensive agents in the Division of Obstetrics and Gynaecology, St Mary's Hospital, London.

PATIENTS AND METHODS

Between January 1970 and December 1973, eight hypertensive women were treated during nine pregnancies using propranolol combined with other hypotensive agents. Over the same period 15 other hypertensive patients were treated with similar drugs excluding propranolol. The clinical details of each case have been reported elsewhere (Lieberman *et al.*, 1977), but the important features are referred to below.

The shortcomings of retrospective analysis are recognized and a method of multivariate statistical analysis has been used to compare fetal outcome in propranolol-treated and non-propranolol-treated cases. Because the treatment groups were not allocated randomly, the analysis took into account other drugs prescribed before and during pregnancy as well as the severity and aetiology of the hypertension in the two groups. If any selection occurred in drug prescription the analysis should minimize its effects on the conclusions reached.

Despite its relative lack of sensitivity, the highest diastolic blood-pressure measured during pregnancy was found to be the best indicator of the degree of hypertension which, along with the maximum excretion of proteinuria per day and the highest level of blood urea, gave an easily recognizable measure of the severity of the hypertensive disorder. Blood uric acid levels were not measured in enough patients to be included. The presence or absence of parenchymal renal disease and birthweight for gestational age and sex related to the fifth centile (Thomson *et al.*, 1968) were included in the analysis as independent variables.

For the purpose of analysis, therefore, fetal outcome was taken as a response to several independent variables of which treatment with propranolol was one. The analysis was then performed by regressing fetal outcome on the measures of treatment, renal disease and severity of hypertension (the logistic transformation was used for fetal outcome, to improve the linearity of its relationship to the independent variables). It resulted in a regression coefficient for each independent variable and a constant term. To assess the importance of any variable in determining fetal outcome the regression equation may be recalculated with that variable omitted. If the variation in fetal outcome accounted for by the first equation is compared with that of the second, the difference reflects the variation due to the omitted variable and thus its contribution to the explanation of observed deaths.

RESULTS

Seven of the nine propranolol-treated pregnancies and three of the 15 pregnancies treated otherwise ended in fetal death. Placental insufficiency was the proven cause in three of the propranolol-treated cases and one of the

46

others whereas the cause was not so easily determined in the remainder. Another two infants died shortly after birth: in neither case had propranolol been prescribed, but in one, labour had to be induced between 28 and 29 weeks' gestation. Labour began spontaneously at 30 weeks in the second and the baby died of atelectasis. None of the 24 fetuses was congenitally abnormal.

Table 4.1

Variable	Coefficient $(+S.E.)$	Variation due to variable $(\chi^2, 1 \text{ d.f.})$	Significance
(Constant term)	$-4\cdot9673 \pm 3\cdot4317$		
Propranolol*	$1\cdot3286 \pm 0\cdot7598$	3·848	$P < 0\cdot05$
Maximum proteinuria/24 hours	$0\cdot3196 \pm 0\cdot2157$	2·895	$P < 0\cdot10$
Maximum diastolic blood-pressure	$0\cdot0291 \pm 0\cdot0260$	1·391	N.S.
Maximum blood urea mg/100 ml	$0\cdot0203 \pm 0\cdot0199$	1·072	N.S.
Renal disease†	$-0\cdot4148 \pm 0\cdot8517$	0·255	N.S.

* Coded 1 if prescribed, 0 otherwise
† Coded 1 if present, 0 otherwise

Table 4.1 shows the results of the multivariate analysis and suggests that within this group of severely hypertensive women only two of the variables were associated to any degree with poor fetal outcome. These were the level of proteinuria and the treatment with propranolol. Table 4.2 shows the perinatal mortality related to aetiology of the hypertension in the two treat-

Table 4.2   Perinatal mortality related to the aetiology of hypertension and treatment*

	Renal disease	Essential hypertension	Polycystic kidney	Renal artery stenosis
Propranolol (with other drugs)	5/6	2/2	—	0/1†
No propranolol (but other drugs)	2/3	3/9	0/2	0/1

* First figure denotes deaths, the second the total number treated
† Combined with coarctation of aorta

ment groups. The diagnosis of renal disease was made before or after the index pregnancy by renal biopsy in five cases, and by intravenous pyelogram and/or renogram in three. It was presumptive in one case.

It can be seen that, despite the lack of significant association between outcome and renal disease in Table 4.1, the majority of patients with renal disease were propranolol-treated and the outcome was bad whatever the treatment. Table 4.3 tends to confirm that there was no trend towards treating patients who had the most marked proteinuria with propranolol.

Pre-eclampsia supervened in two propranolol-treated and in three non-propranolol cases: no babies survived. The mean maximum blood-pressure

Table 4.3 Fetal outcome related to maximum level of proteinuria and treatment*

	Nil	*Less than 2 g/day*	*2 g/day or more*
Propranolol (with other drugs)	2/3	2/2	3/4
No propranolol (but other drugs)	1/7	0/3	4/5

* The first figure denotes perinatal deaths, the second the total number in each group

readings in the whole propranolol and non-propranolol-treated groups were 190/110 and 185/120 mmHg respectively. The degree of control of hypertension is an important factor but it proved hard to quantify. As propranolol may have been used in cases difficult to control otherwise, reasons for its prescription were examined. In three cases it appears to have been used because it was a new, effective therapy and in the same number it was prescribed because hypertension had been difficult to control outwith pregnancy. There was no obvious indication in two cases and one patient became pregnant while taking it (it was stopped at 20 weeks' gestation). In eight women it was not prescribed when the blood-pressure patterns were similar to those which had otherwise seemed to justify its use. Control was adequate in six women without altering their pre-pregnant therapy which did not include propranolol. The hypertension was so fulminating in one case that control was difficult whatever was prescribed. It does not seem, therefore, that propranolol was prescribed more often when hypertension was difficult to control.

Because nine hypotensive agents had been administered in various combinations in the 24 pregnancies, no reliable estimate of the effect of each drug could be obtained. Pentolinium, clonidine, and intermittent hydrallazine had been prescribed for so few patients (one, one and three respectively) that they were excluded from the analysis. The other six hypotensive agents used were reserpine, debrisoquine, guanethidine, bethanidine, methyldopa and amiloride hydrochloride (with hydrochlorothiazide). Treatment with drugs other than propranolol was measured by the total number prescribed before and during pregnancy.

Twelve patients became pregnant whilst on hypotensive therapy including three on propranolol. Nine of these babies survived, the two in the propranolol group being its only survivors. In one of these propranolol was discontinued at 20 weeks' gestation. Of the 12 cases in which hypotensive therapy was begun during pregnancy only three babies survived. Six of the nine babies that died were in the propranolol group.

In two cases intrauterine death occurred within 48 hours of the commencement of propranolol (at 29 and 34 weeks respectively). In a further four cases the fetus succumbed 10 days, 4, 5, and 18 weeks later respectively. The median maximum dose of propranolol was 160 mg/day, the range being 80 to 960 mg/day.

In all cases save one in which drugs other than propranolol were used the prescriptions began early in pregnancy and continued throughout. This applied whether or not the baby survived. The exceptional case was so fulminating due to superadded pre-eclampsia that reserpine and intermittent hydrallazine failed to produce any benefit and a stillbirth resulted.

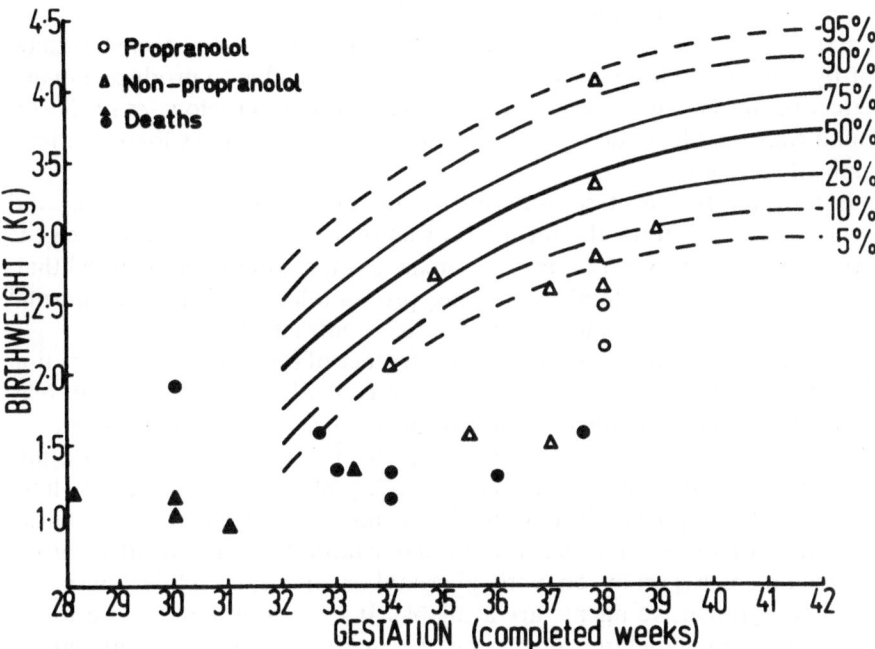

Figure 4.1 Fetal outcome related to birthweight for gestational age

Figure 4.1 shows that, regardless of therapy, no babies survived from the eight pregnancies which ended before 34 weeks' gestation. The four deaths from this gestation occurred in the propranolol group. There was no association between treatment and birthweight or gestation, but of those babies who died the propranolol group were heavier and older than the 'other drugs' group. Thus increased growth retardation did not seem to contribute significantly to the excess perinatal loss in the propranolol group.

DISCUSSION

Propranolol may, therefore, decrease the chances of fetal survival when used to treat severely hypertensive pregnant women in whom placental insufficiency is already a hazard. The lack of adverse effects reported by Turner *et al.* (1968) in the management of hypertrophic obstructive cardiomyopathy during pregnancy may be because the placentae were functioning normally. Gladstone *et al.* (1975) and Fiddler (1974) have linked the use of propranolol with intrauterine growth retardation, intrapartum asphyxia, neonatal brady-cardia, and neonatal hypoglycaemia. Tunstall (1969) and Reed (1974) have, in different circumstances, reported inhibition of respiration in the neonate associated with propranolol administration and it is known that it crosses the placenta (Masuoka and Hansson, 1967).

Experimental evidence too tends to incriminate beta-adrenergic blockade for by using it Rudolph and Heymann (1973) were able to produce a major reduction in fetal heart rate and in cardiac output. Truelove *et al.* (1973) found that the blockade lasted between two and three times longer in fetal lambs than in ewes.

But by far the most serious reports are by Joelsson *et al.* (1972) and Renou *et al.* (1969) for the former showed that beta-blockade rendered the fetus less capable of responding to anoxia and the latter demonstrated that, besides reducing the fetal heart rate, propranolol abolished the normal increase in fetal heart rate in response to a contraction.

Adamsons has suggested that 'in the presence of optimal fetal oxygenation the effects of beta-sympathetic blockade are small and perhaps of no rele-vance, while they become conspicuous in the presence of fetal asphyxia'.

Thus, the experimental evidence and the results of the present study suggest that propranolol may limit the ability of the growth retarded fetus to respond to hypoxia. Despite the shortcomings of a retrospective analysis it is, therefore, suggested that propranolol cannot be recommended for use in pregnancy hypertension with placental insufficiency while alternative effective hypotensive agents are available. It is even doubted if the use of beta-adrenergic blocking agents can be made the subject of an ethical prospective study in such patients.

References

Adamsons, K. (1973). Personal communication

Feitelson, P. J. and Lindheimer, M. D. (1972). Management of hypertensive gravidae. *J. Reprod. Med.*, **8**, 111

Fiddler, G. I. (1974). Propranolol and pregnancy. *Lancet*, ii, 722

Gladstone, G. R., Hordof, A. and Gersony, W. M. (1975). Propranolol administration during pregnancy. Effects on the fetus. *J. Pediatr.*, **86**, 962

Hans, S. F. and Kopelman, H. (1964). Methyldopa in treatment of severe toxaemia of pregnancy. *Br. Med. J.*, **1**, 736

Holland, O. B. and Kaplan, N. M. (1976). Propranolol in the treatment of hypertension. *N. Engl. J. Med.*, **294** (17), 930

Joelsson, I., Barton, M. D., Daniel, S., James, S. and Adamsons, K. (1972). The response of the unanaesthetized sheep fetus to sympathomimetic amines and adrenergic blocking agents. *Am. J. Obstet Gynecol.*, **114**, 43

Kincaid-Smith, P., Bullen, M. and Mills, J. (1966). Prolonged use of methyldopa in severe hypertension in pregnancy. *Br. Med. J.*, **1**, 274

Leather, H. M., Humphreys, D. M., Baker, P. and Chadd, M. A. (1968). A controlled trial of hypotensive agents in hypertension in pregnancy. *Lancet*, **ii**, 488

Lieberman, B. A., Stirrat, G. M., Beard, R. W., Cohen, S. and Pinker, G. D. (1977). The possible adverse effects of propranolol on the fetus in women with severe hypertension. (In press)

Masuoka, D. and Hansson, E. (1967). Autoradiographic distribution studies of adrenergic blocking agents II. 14C propranolol, a beta-receptor type blocker. *Acta Pharmacol. Toxicol.*, **25**, 447

Prichard, B. N. C. and Gillam, P. M. S. (1969). Treatment of hypertension with propranolol. *Br. Med. J.*, **1**, 7

Redman, C. W. G., Beilin, L. J., Bonnar, J. and Ounsted, M. K. (1976). Fetal outcome in trial of antihypertensive treatment in pregnancy. *Lancet*, **ii**, 753

Reed, R. L. (1974). Propranolol therapy throughout pregnancy. *Anaes. Analg.*, **53**, 214

Renou, P., Newman, W. and Wood, C. (1969). Autonomic control of fetal heart rate. *Am. J. Obstet. Gynecol.*, **105**, 949

Rudolph, A. M. and Heymann, M. A. (1973). Control of the foetal circulation. In *Fetal and Neonatal Physiology*, p. 93. (Cambridge: Cambridge University Press)

Thomson, A. M., Billewicz, W. Z. and Hytten, F. E. (1968). The assessment of fetal growth. *J. Obstet. Gynaecol. Br. Commonw.*, **75**, 903

Truelove, J. F., van Petten, G. R. and Willes, R. F. (1973). Action of several β-adrenoceptor blocking drugs in the pregnant sheep and fetus. *Br. J. Pharmacol.*, **47**, 161

Tunstall, M. E. (1969). The effect of propranolol on the onset of breathing at birth. *Br. J. Anaesth.*, **41**, 792

Turner, G. M., Oakley, C. M. and Dixon, H. G. (1968). Management of pregnancy complicated by hypertrophic obstructive cardiomyopathy. *Br. Med. J.*, **4**, 281

Discussion

de Swiet: Was there a correlation between proteinuria and propranolol therapy in these patients?

Stirrat: There was no correlation between taking propranolol and proteinuria. In analysing these data each variable was considered individually. Proteinuria was a significant predictor of fetal death, as was propranolol therapy.

de Swiet: May it not be that the patients with bad proteinuria were more likely to be put on propranolol and that the cause of fetal death was the severity of the illness and not the treatment to which they were exposed?

Stirrat: I do not think that this was the case. We looked at the reason for initiating treatment in all cases. In three cases propranolol was used because of its known renin suppressing action. In a further two cases there appeared to be no clear indication for the drug and these patients did not have severe proteinuria. In a further three propranolol was added because the hypertension was difficult to control.

5
The Management of Hypertension in the Pregnant Woman*

P. J. LEWIS, M. de SWIET, G. V. P. CHAMBERLAIN and C. J. BULPITT

OBJECTIVES

In 1975 a postal survey of obstetricians in the British Isles was undertaken to discover how women with hypertension were managed during pregnancy. This study was initiated as part of the planning of a prospective investigation of whether antihypertensive drug therapy during pregnancy in women with pre-existing hypertension can improve prognosis for the fetus.

In designing such a study an important consideration was that the control group of women should receive such treatment as was generally accepted as the best currently available. The treated group could then receive this treatment plus the drug or drugs being investigated. An obvious initial problem in mounting such an investigation was to decide which treatment was generally accepted as the best currently available. This was the primary objective of conducting the survey.

BACKGROUND TO THE SURVEY

As perinatal mortality due to avoidable causes continues to fall attention focuses on more intransigent causes of fetal loss such as fetal malformation and maternal hypertension. Women whose arterial blood-pressure is elevated, either as a result of some primary condition such as renal disease, or simply because they fall into the upper part of the population distribution of arterial pressure, the so-called 'essential hypertensives', are at increased risk

* This study was supported by a grant from Merck Sharp and Dhome Ltd.

of having an unsuccessful pregnancy (Butler and Bonham, 1963; Tervila *et al.*, 1973). The fetus may grow poorly, die *in utero* or be delivered prematurely. It is likely that these adverse consequences of raised blood-pressure are due to impaired placental perfusion which may occur chronically during the second and third trimesters of pregnancy and acutely if the syndrome of pre-eclampsia supervenes (Dixon *et al.*, 1963).

Treatment of women whose arterial pressure is raised from the beginning of pregnancy is a matter of controversy. Traditionally women with hypertension have been discouraged from pregnancy especially if they have renal impairment. Once pregnant the usual regime employed has depended largely on bed-rest, reduced activity, sedative drugs and premature delivery of the child (Dewhurst, 1976).

Antihypertensive drugs have been eschewed by most obstetricians on the grounds that the raised arterial pressure was necessary for the perfusion of the diseased placenta and that lowering the blood-pressure would further impair fetal nutrition. This belief is reminiscent of the reaction of physicians to antihypertensive treatment when it was first introduced into general medicine. In the event, hypertension did not prove 'essential' for the perfusion of the brain and kidneys, and lowering the blood-pressure diminished the incidence of stroke and uraemia rather than precipitating these events. However, in the case of the placenta autoregulation is more rudimentary and there is some experimental work to suggest that placental underperfusion may occur when blood-pressure is reduced (de Swiet and Hoffbrand, 1971). In human pregnancy there is little indication that lowering blood-pressure lowers placental perfusion.

METHODS

A multiple choice questionnaire was devised and mailed to all fellows and members of the Royal College of Obstetricians and Gynaecologists who were listed as resident in the British Isles (UK and Eire). Included with the questionnaire was a reply paid envelope. If no reply had been received within 3 months a second questionnaire was sent.

The questionnaire consisted of a 12-page booklet accompanied by an explanatory letter listing the aims of the survey and asking that questions be answered as if they related to the obstetrician's own practice. Most of the questions consisted of a stem which presented a precise case history; the respondents were asked to indicate which of an exhaustive series of alternative treatments they would employ.

RESULTS
Response to the survey

A total of 1987 questionnaires were mailed: 1314 to members and 673 to fellows of the College. 36 questionnaires were returned as the addressee had moved and no forwarding address was known. A total of 1484 replies were received, a gross response rate of 76%. Of the respondents 391 indicated that they had retired or had not engaged in clinical obstetrics during the preceding 12 months. Replies from these individuals were not analysed in the survey and hence the population studied was 1093 individuals who replied to the questionnaire and who were in active practice either in the UK or Eire. Of the 1093 individuals 808 were practising in England, 129 were practising in Scotland, 52 in Wales, 41 in Northern Ireland and 63 in Eire.

Replies

Ethics of a prospective control trial of antihypertensive drug treatment in pregnancy

Since an important primary motive in making this survey was to prepare for a prospective investigation the use of antihypertensive drugs during pregnancy it was decided to take the opportunity to ask obstetricians whether they considered such an investigation was warranted or ethical. The question asked was: 'Supposing a randomized control trial was proposed to compare the effects of antihypertensive drug treatment with placebo treatment during pregnancy in women with pre-existing hypertension. Do you think that:

(i) This trial would be unnecessary since it is established that antihypertensive drugs do not improve fetal outcome?

or

(ii) Unnecessary since it is established that antihypertensive drugs do improve fetal outcome?

or

(iii) Desirable because the matter is not clearly decided?

19% replied (i), 7% replied (ii) and 69% replied (iii). A second question asked at what diastolic pressure it would be ethical to withdraw women on placebo and place them on treatment. 36% thought that women should be withdrawn if their diastolic blood-pressure rose to 100 mmHg and a further 44% thought they should be withdrawn if their diastolic blood-pressure rose to 110 mmHg.

Management of hypertension with and without renal impairment

The following case was presented: A woman of 28 is found to have consistently raised blood-pressure at the 16th week of her first pregnancy. Supposing the blood-pressure was either 140/90 mmHg or 170/110 mmHg what would be your immediate management of this patient? In a further rider to this question the patient was stated to have either a normal plasma urea or a plasma urea of 75 mg/100 ml. These permutations of blood-pressure and renal function gave four clinical situations. Table 5.1 shows the immediate management chosen by the respondents.

Table 5.1   Immediate management of a woman of 28 at 16 weeks of pregnancy with hypertension and renal impairment. Figures are the percentage of respondents who would employ the management indicated

Blood-pressure (mmHg)	140/95	170/110	140/95	170/110
Plasma urea (mg/100 ml)	<20	<20	75	75
Admit to hospital	43	96	95	98
Consider terminating this pregnancy	0	28	42	73
Insist on bed-rest	41	82	77	89
Treat with an antihypertensive drug	13	73	32	77

Termination of pregnancy was considered in these four cases by a surprisingly high proportion of respondents. Figure 5.1 shows a further analysis of this result where the replies to this question were further analysed according to the year of specialist qualification of the respondent. It is evident that

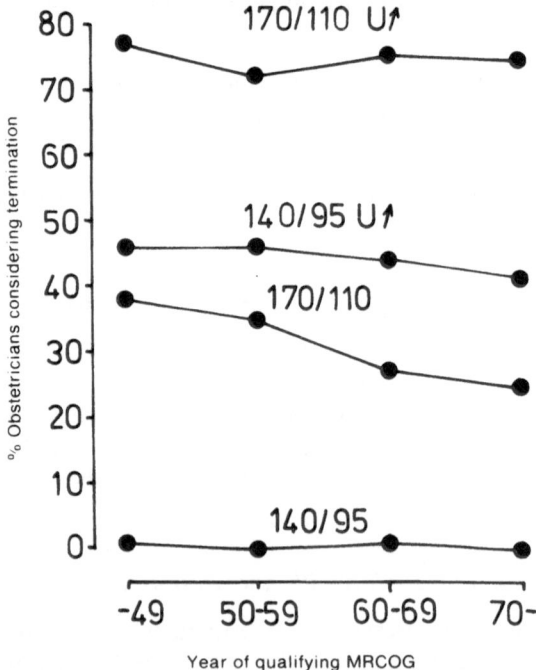

Figure 5.1   Percentage of obstetricians in active practice who would consider termination of pregnancy in a 28-year-old primipara with raised blood-pressure at 16 weeks' gestation and a normal or raised blood urea, according to year of specialist qualification of the respondent

the clinical situation of the patient is a much more important determinant of the reply than the seniority of the obstetrician. There is nevertheless a tendency for more senior obstetricians to consider termination of pregnancy more readily in these women with hypertension with or without impaired renal function.

A further question was asked concerning drug treatment in these cases. A choice of immediate treatment with either diazepam, a barbiturate, a diuretic, an antihypertensive or no drug was offered. Respondents were asked to choose the one treatment they thought most appropriate. Figure 5.2 shows the proportion of respondents choosing each treatment according to the severity of the hypertension and renal impairment. While few obstetricians chose to use an antihypertensive drug at a blood-pressure of 140/95 mmHg most respondents would use this in either case if the blood-pressure were 170/110 mmHg. Conversely the proportion of respondents using no drug or sedative therapy decreases as the arterial pressure is increased.

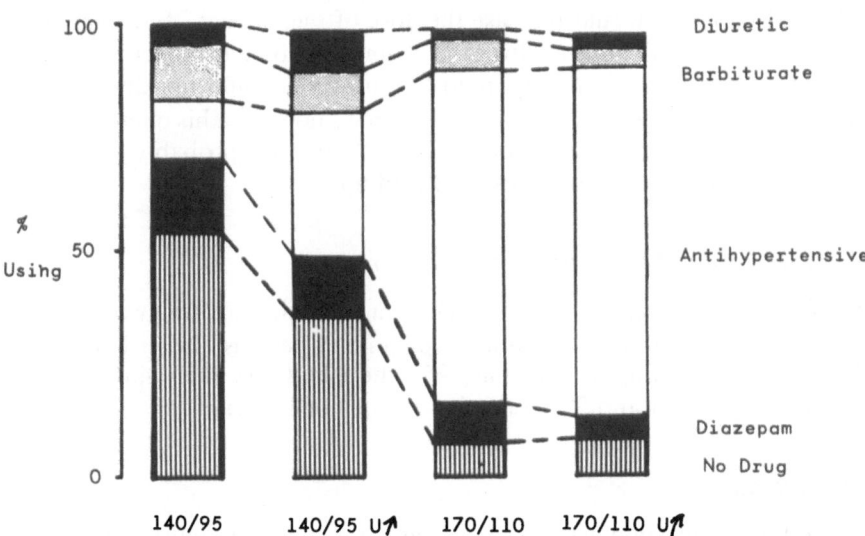

Figure 5.2 Drug treatment chosen for a 28-year-old primipara with raised blood-pressure at 16 weeks' gestation and a normal or raised blood urea. Histograms show the percentage of obstetricians choosing each treatment

Essential hypertension already on treatment

The following case question was posed: 'A woman of 28 is known to have essential hypertension and has been treated for 4 years with methyldopa (Aldomet) and a diuretic. She has normal renal function and is in the 16th week of her first pregnancy with a blood-pressure on treatment of 130/80 mmHg'. The first question asked was whether the respondent would stop or continue these drugs. 13% would stop both drugs, 22% would stop the diuretic, 1% would stop the methyldopa and 63% would continue both drugs. A second rider asked what would be the anticipated date of delivery of this patient. 1% favoured 34–35 weeks, 14% favoured 36–37 weeks, 78% favoured 38–39 weeks. Only 5% would allow the patient to go to term.

Severe hypertension with renal impairment

The following question was asked: 'A woman of 28 is in the 12th week of her first pregnancy. At the age of 16 she was treated for severe hypertension, secondary to glomerulonephritis. She has been on antihypertensive drugs since that time and has diminished renal function with a blood urea of 75 mg/100 ml. Her blood-pressure is 140/95 mmHg on treatment. Would you urge termination of pregnancy? 28% of the respondents said that they would urge termination of pregnancy. Concerning the drug treatment, 96% of respondents said that they would continue the antihypertensive drugs and 17% said that they would increase the dose of these drugs. A further rider asked: 'Would you plan to deliver this woman as soon as the fetus is viable (i.e. has a satisfactory amniotic fluid lecithin/sphyngomyelin ratio) even if her blood-pressure were well controlled?' 76% said yes to this question while 21% said no. A further question asked: 'Would you probably deliver by Caesarian section?' 66% said yes, 31% said no.

Natural history of essential hypertension

The following question was asked: 'Do you think that treating women with essential hypertensive drugs during pregnancy lessens the risk of their developing pre-eclamptic toxaemia?' 25% thought it very likely, 45% thought it probably did not and 29% said that it was not known.

Drugs used

The following question was asked: 'A patient with moderately severe hypertension becomes pregnant while taking antihypertensive drugs. Her physician wishes her to continue such treatment for the majority of the antenatal period. Which drug, if any, would you be quite happy for the patient to continue taking up until labour and which would you prefer stopped or changed?' A list of antihypertensive drugs was given and for each the respondent was invited to say whether the drug represented no problem, whether he would prefer it changed or whether he had no experience with the drug. Many obstetricians said they had no experience of propranolol, clonidine or bethanidine. Almost all obstetricians said they had experience with diuretic or methyldopa. The proportion of respondents having experience of particular antihypertensive drugs in pregnancy is shown related to seniority of the obstetrician in Figure 5.3. It can be seen that recently qualified obstetricians were more familiar with propranolol. clonidine and bethanidine than obstetricians who qualified earlier. Amongst those who

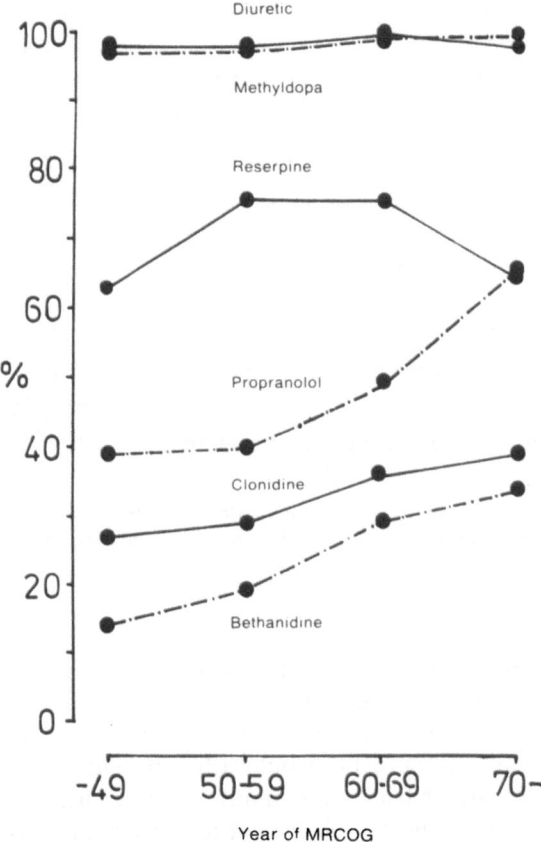

Figure 5.3 Percentage of obstetricians having experience of particular antihypertensive drugs in pregnancy according to year of specialist qualification

said they had experience of the drugs, the proportion expressing approval or disapproval for their use in pregnancy differed with individual drugs. Figure 5.4 illustrates these results.

Methyldopa and diuretic were the drugs most approved of for use in pregnancy, methyldopa being approved by over 90% of all obstetricians familiar with its use. Debrisoquine and bethanidine were approved by just over half of respondents. Reserpine and propranolol were thought to present no problem by one-third of those having experience in their use.

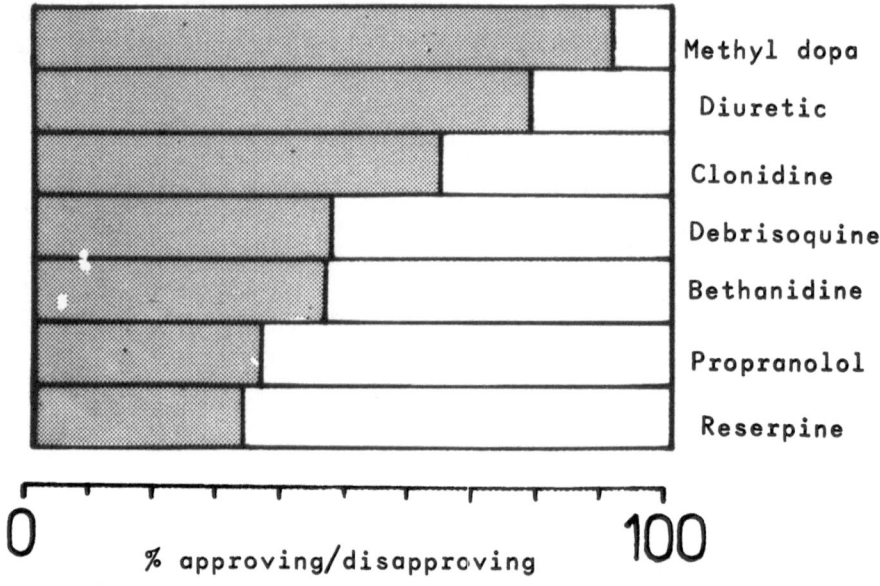

Figure 5.4 Percentage of obstetricians having experience of an antihypertensive drug in pregnancy approving or disapproving of the drug for use throughout pregnancy.

DISCUSSION

We were very appreciative that such a high proportion of obstetricians contributed to this survey. Even if it were assumed that all 467 obstetricians who did not reply were in active practice, which is most unlikely, then our 1093 respondents in active practice would still represent 70% of all practising obstetricians in the British Isles, a very impressive proportion. This completeness of coverage adds considerable weight to our conclusions and makes it very likely that our results do give a good indication of how women with hypertension are managed during pregnancy.

The most striking conclusion which can be drawn from our data is that pregnancy in a woman with hypertension is very pessimistically regarded. We did not canvass this opinion directly but it can be inferred from the high proportion of respondents who considered termination of pregnancy in the cases presented and who urged termination of pregnancy in the case of a woman with severe hypertension and renal impairment. Since the clinical features of hypertension and raised blood urea would be recurrent this amounts to a proscription of pregnancy in women with severe hypertension and renal disease. This pessimistic attitude is presumably related to a clinical experience of poor outcome in these cases. It certainly indicates that ways of improving the fetal outcome in such cases are genuinely required.

A second conclusion which emerges is that there is a broad consensus on how women with hypertension are managed at present. In 18 out of 22 questions posed concerning case management, 70% or more of respondents gave the same opinions. The questions where there was a greater difference of opinion were related to management of the more mild cases of hypertension and also on the use of antihypertensive drugs.

In general the respondents were conservative in their approach to antihypertensive drugs. If a woman presented already on antihypertensive treatment then this would be continued. If a woman presented with hypertension then respondents were reluctant to initiate treatment. If a patient on antihypertensive drugs presented with an elevated blood-pressure during pregnancy the respondents would prefer not to increase the dose of drugs. All these replies indicate that obstetricians are uncertain of the potential benefit or harm of the treatment to the fetus and the majority of respondents admitted this directly by supporting the idea that a prospective therapeutic trial should be mounted. It is of interest that of those who consider the question of antihypertensive drugs settled, more than twice as many consider it proven that the drugs are of no value to the fetus. However, the fact that most obstetricians would think it unethical to withhold antihypertensive drugs if the mother's diastolic blood pressure rose to 110 mmHg implies that they consider there is a definite hazard at this level of pressure. Presumably in view of the uncertainty of the value of the drugs to the fetus the dangers of withholding treatment at this degree of hypertension are thought to be maternal.

The replies given on the experience of and approval of various antihypertensive drugs for use during pregnancy were very much as had been expected; experience was largely with the major drugs, methyldopa, diuretics and hydrallazine. These drugs were thought to present no problem whereas two-thirds of respondents thought that propranolol should be changed to another drug during pregnancy. In view of the opinions on the use of beta-blockers expressed elsewhere in this volume it is in fact surprising that such a large number of obstetricians have had experience of propranolol in pregnancy. Indeed 184 obstetricians replied that they had experience of propranolol and thought its use presented no problem during pregnancy.

We may conclude there is general agreement amongst practising obstetricians in the British Isles that the management of hypertension in women who become pregnant is unsatisfactory; the outlook for successful pregnancy in these women is poor and the role of antihypertensive drug treatment is ill defined. Whether such hypertensive women receive drugs during pregnancy depends primarily on whether they are already receiving them or whether the hypertension is diagnosed for the first time when the patient becomes pregnant. Few more direct calls for a prospective investigation into a therapeutic problem in pregnancy can have been issued.

References

Butler, N. R. and Bonham, D. G. (1963). Perinatal mortality: first report of British Perinatal mortality Survey. Edinburgh

Dewhurst, C. J. (ed.) (1976). *Integrated Obstetrics and Gynaecology for Postgraduates.* 2nd ed. (Oxford: Blackwell Scientific Publications)

Dixon, H. G., Browne, J. C. M. and Darcy, D. A. (1963). Choriodecidual and myometrial blood flow. *Lancet*, **ii**, 369

Greiss, F. C. (1967). A clinical concept of uterine blood flow during pregnancy. *Obstet. Gynecol.*, **30**, 595

de Swiet, M. and Hoffbrand, B. I. (1971). Effect of bethanidine on placental blood flow in conscious rabbits. *Am. J. Obstet. Gynecol.*, **111**, 374

Tervila, L., Goecke, C. and Timonen, S. (1973). Estimation of gestosis of pregnancy (EPH-gestosis). *Acta Obstet. Gynecol. Scand.*, **52**, 235

Discussion

Niven, P. A. R., Bristol: I found some of these questions very difficult to answer. For example, it is impossible to predict at the 12th week of pregnancy whether one would wish to deliver a woman at the 36th, 37th or 40th week of gestation. This decision must depend on how the pregnancy has progressed and in particular how the fetus has grown. Did many obstetricians comment on the difficulty in replying to some of these questions?

Lewis: I should like to make the point first of all that the questionnaire as sent out represents something like a tenth draft. After designing the questions we did a pilot survey to get comments of obstetricians as to the comprehensibility of the questionnaire. I agree that one major difficulty was asking obstetricians to take decisions on their likely management ahead of time. However, in the case of the question which you cited we wish to know whether obstetricians anticipated that a well-controlled hypertensive pregnancy would go to term or whether even in well-controlled cases they would be unhappy to see this happen.

With regard to the number of obstetricians who made comments as to the structure of the questionnaire, we did have a section for free comment. 45% of those who replied wrote comments and many of these related to specific questions in the questionnaire rather than making general comments about the management of hypertension in pregnancy. Some obstetricians made the general point that it was impossible to categorize patients and that each individual case must be treated on its own merit. I must say that I profoundly disagree with this attitude towards medical treatment. It is only by categorizing patients in a rigid way and applying standard treatments that therapeutic decisions can be evaluated. Several obstetricians wrote that it would be virtually impossible to arrange a randomized control trial on the effects of anti-hypertensive drug treatment during pregnancy because truly comparable groups could not be selected. This attitude is probably widespread because obstetrics is a branch of medicine in which very few randomized control trials are carried out and indeed many of the treatments in current use have never been rigorously evaluated. However, medicine is either a science or an art, if it is a science then we should try to evaluate our treatments in a scientific way.

Dollery: I think I can summarize after this last paper on hypertension what we have heard of the relative values of different treatment regimens in the following way:

Rest and sedation seem to be very good, methyldopa seems to be good, diuretics seem to be maybe and propranolol seems to be bad. It appears we are very long on opinion and pretty short on evidence in favour of most of those statements. In fact the only statement which was really strongly supported by evidence was the one concerned with methyldopa from Dr Beilin. And so perhaps a thing we should focus on first of all is the question about propranolol. Is there anybody in the audience who wants to take issue with what has been said or record of more favourable experiences with propranolol? If not, then let us ask the speakers about this apparent difference between propranolol and methyldopa. Professor Dawes, you said that you were concerned about effects on catecholamines responses with propranolol but there is data in patients treated long term with methyldopa showing they have a plasma noradrenaline concentration about one half what it is in people treated with diuretics for example. If catechecholamine responses are so important to the fetus surely methyldopa also should be harmful to it?

Dawes: My difficulty about this is that I do not really understand how methyldopa works and I think that that opinion is shared by a lot of pharmacologists. However, if catecholamines still act in its presence and if catecholamines are still released then obviously it is not going to be nearly so dangerous as propranolol. There is another consideration which I think ought to be born in mind. This is that the great majority of the animal experiments that have been done with these drugs have been short term and you are now talking about a clinical situation where these drugs are used for weeks at a time. There is one other nice theoretical point. It is widely believed that during the last half of gestation the central nervous organization is set which determines subsequent behaviour postnatally. How drugs might affect this organization is at present highly speculative, but it is something we have got to be aware of in the future. I am not trying to create unnecessary fears but on a purely factual basis we do not have the information.

Dollery: Dr Beilin, can we come back to you because you have done a study which has shown the benefit of methyldopa treatment. I would like to know what you think about propranolol and I would like to put a point to you. One of the things that concerns me in the rather theoretical discourses against propranolol is I can remember exactly the same kind of points being made in adult non-pregnant medicine in relation to beta-blocking drugs. For example, I can remember people saying it would be very dangerous if somebody had a myocardial infarction while on a beta-blocker because the heart would be in a very unfavourable situation being no longer able to respond to sympathetic drive and raise the cardiac output. However, there are now convincing randomized controlled trials in the literature saying that if you give beta-blocking drugs to patients in the 2 years after a myocardial infarction you in fact reduce mortality significantly rather than increasing it. So I think that one has got to be very careful about theoretical arguments with beta-blockers. Do you have any experience with propranolol and what is your opinion about it in pregnancy?

Beilin: We do not have any experience with propranolol but what you said I would have said had you given me the chance. I agree with you that I have had a very much *deju vu* feeling when Professor Dawes was propounding the hazards of propranolol on the basis of experimental data. These were exactly the arguments that we used against the use of propranolol in non-pregnant patients and I think what we really need to know is precisely how the fetus dies in pre-eclampsia, really whether it is dying as a result of ventricular fibrillation for example rather than anoxia. This is something that I suppose might be possible to learn with fetal electrocardiography in the human and much easier to learn in animals. If the fetus were to die in ventricular fibrillation then still on a purely theoretical basis one might be a little more encouraged to use a drug like propranolol which might protect against such an event. I think the difficulty as you pin-point, is knowing whether it is justified to do any form of clinical trial with propranolol given that there are other antihypertensive drugs that one can use in pregnancy and that unlike the non-pregnant situation this whole condition has a very limited time course. I would rather see more animal data particularly on primates, particularly on non-anaesthetized primates on the effects of different beta-blockers on cardiac function.

Dollery: Can I ask you Professor Dawes, whether it is known if beta-blockers given throughout pregnancy to animals affect the weight of the heart and therefore the weight of the whole fetus?

Dawes: No. As I was careful to say no-one has given prolonged propranolol treatment in either monkeys or sheep. If I can come back to the most important point of all, I think, of course you are perfectly correct in the analogy that you draw with the adult. However, in the fetus the most important hazard is hypoxia. The fetus has a PO_2 of 24. If any of us here had a PO_2 of 24 we would be unconscious. In fact there are a lot of infants with a PO_2 which is very much less than that and they can survive *in utero* for a limited period of time with a PO_2 of 10, so it is an entirely different situation that we are discussing here and that is really why I am so sceptical about beta-blockers in this regard.

Mucklow, J., London: Is there any reason to suggest that methyldopa given in the first 12 weeks of pregnancy has a teratogenic effect?

Beilin: In the trial I reported the women all started treatment after the 12th week of pregnancy so we cannot help there. Our practise had been that if a woman is on methyldopa and becomes pregnant and the hypertension is not severe, we prefer to stop the drug until after the 12th week of pregnancy.

Dollery: There must have been quite a few hypertensive women on methyldopa who did not declare themselves to be pregnant until after that time. As far as I know no-one has reported teratogenicity. Mr Hawkins, can you comment?

Hawkins: I think the only evidence of a teratogenic effect has been the generation of a positive Coombs in the baby.

McDevitt, D. J., Belfast: I would like to ask Dr Beilin two questions. He said that in the methyldopa group there was no effect of treatment on birthweight or placental weight. I would like to ask him how he thinks methyldopa improves the fetal position in hypertension? The second point is a more general one which I think has been raised in comments by various people. If I understood Dr Lewis's questionnaire rightly, propranolol is already being used perhaps quite widely in women with hypertension in pregnancy. In view of that is it correct that people should question the ethics of doing trials of propranolol in the treatment of hypertension in pregnancy? It would surely be better that it be demonstrated that propranolol is indeed harmful rather that people should go on using it without reliable information.

Beilin: Perhaps I can take the last question first. I think the basis for doing any trial is to show benefit whether it is in pregnant or non-pregnant patients. Unless one has at least some theoretical reasons why a treatment might be doing good rather than doing harm, there is no point in using it. Possibly one should spend time trying to educate people as to why not to use it. But the problem is that the vast majority of patients on whom propranolol is used all have mild to moderate hypertension and will have successful pregnancies anyway. This means that the people who are using it are not going to accumulate the evidence that will tell them whether it is doing harm or good in the few who develop severe pre-eclampsia or the few who lose their babies.

The question of how methyldopa has a beneficial effect on fetal outcome is a difficult one. I do not really know. I can speculate that since methyldopa affects the endocrine system, for example in the non-pregnant patient it will elevate prolactin levels, then some endocrine effect might be responsible. The sympathetic nervous system affects uterine tone and again methyldopa might have effects there.

Part 2
Cardiovascular Therapy

6
Heart Disease, Parturition and Antibiotic Prophylaxis

ROSALINDE HURLEY

The relative incidence of congenital and rheumatic heart disease in obstetric practice is changing. Hamilton (1947) recorded chronic rheumatic heart disease in 93% of 1335 pregnant cardiac patients; miscellaneous cardiovascular diseases, including syphilis, occurred in 1·8%, and 5·2% had congenital cardiovascular defects. The ratio of 1:20 for congenital and rheumatic heart disease was also observed by Szekely and Snaith (1974), during the 10-year period between 1942 and 1951, but changed to 1:3 in the decade 1962–1971. The decrease of rheumatic heart disease in the community is reflected in obstetric practice (Hurley, 1972) and early palliative and corrective surgery results in an absolute increase in the number of women with congenital heart disease who reach childbearing age.

Estimates of the incidence of congenital heart anomalies have varied from 0·5/1000 to 21·0/1000 total births, but errors including inaccuracy of diagnosis and lack of follow-up of children who show no evidence of congenital heart disease in infancy suggest that the given figures fall short of the true total. An average of 6–8/1000 live births is generally accepted (Campbell, 1968; 1973). Szekely and Snaith record atrial and ventricular septal defect, ductus arteriosus, pulmonary and aortic stenosis, and coarctation of the aorta as the lesions most frequently encountered in pregnant women in their practice. Cardiac surgery is performed rarely during pregnancy, but both open and closed cardiac surgery are feasible, although the latter carries a risk (Copeland *et al.*, 1963) to mother and fetus. Together with cardio-circulatory failure, infective endocarditis is the main complication of congenital heart disease during pregnancy. In patients who have been subject to cardiac surgery, the valve prosthesis can become infected and less common causative organisms have been documented more often than streptococci in such cases (Clarkson and Barret-Boyes, 1970; Edwards, 1973).

The prevalence of rheumatic heart disease in the child population has been estimated many times and the incidence has varied from 0·2 to 4·5%. The incidence rises as adolescence is approached, so that Keith, Rowe and Vlad (1967) found that by 14 years of age, the rate had risen to 150/100 000 population. There has been a marked decline in the mortality of the disease in childhood, so that it has fallen from being the second leading cause of death in infancy and childhood to seventh place. Both the primary incidence and severity, and the recurrence rate of rheumatic fever have been falling in recent years. Thus Wilson noted that the decline in rheumatic fever recurrence rate began about 1937 and continued until 1956 at a rate of 0·4% per year. The epidemiology of rheumatic fever and rheumatic carditis is complex, and involves not only the haemolytic streptococcus with its well-attested cyclical variation in virulence, but also the rheumatic response of the host to infection, socioeconomic conditions, and the use of antibiotics and steroids. Recurrence of rheumatic fever, with risk of further damage to the heart, and infective endocarditis are complications of rheumatic heart disease that are, probably, averted by the use of prophylactic antibiotics. Either may occur during pregnancy.

Infective endocarditis is more common in males, and is uncommon in pure mitral stenosis, which is by far the most common lesion encountered during pregnancy. However, it was observed in the past, sometimes in the course of puerperal sepsis, and its incidence was, presumably, reduced by the introduction of aseptic methods into obstetric practice. Acute bacterial endocarditis can occur in a pregnant woman with previously normal heart, as part of a general septicaemia. Occurring, as it usually does, in women with valvar disease of the heart, the onset of infective endocarditis may be insidious. The presenting symptoms and signs are variable and early diagnosis may be difficult. This is especially so during pregnancy. Blood culture may be negative (Hayward, 1960) despite clinical features that are virtually diagnostic and even despite postmortem confirmation of the disease. Endocarditis with negative blood culture carries a worse prognosis than that in which the causative microbe can be isolated; Cates and Christie (1951) reported that 52% of 408 patients with positive blood cultures recovered on penicillin therapy, compared with 18% of 34 patients with negative blood cultures. If endocarditis is suspected, therapy should not be postponed more than 48 hours, and if blood cultures are repeatedly sterile, a special regimen of therapy may be required (Keith et al., 1967).

At the Boston Lying-In Hospital, Hamilton (1947) recorded that 20% of maternal deaths among cardiac patients were ascribable to endocarditis, and, before penicillin, accounted for a third of maternal deaths in those with otherwise favourable rheumatic heart disease. All the women he treated, even two treated with penicillin, were dead when he wrote his report, and of 17 women treated elsewhere with penicillin, 53% were dead 5 months after delivery. The fetal mortality was 24%. Pedowitz and Hellman (1953) reported a maternal mortality of 14%. Burwell and Metcalfe (1958) suggest that infective endocarditis is a disappearing disease during pregnancy, and, clearly, with so high a potential mortality, it is well that it is so. Mendelson (1960) treated four pregnant patients successfully, and Szekely and Snaith (1974) treated six, although early heart failure developed in three. Prophylaxis against infective endocarditis during pregnancy and parturition is, of course, widely used, and may account for the low incidence.

Using the figures of Barnes (1970) and Szekely and Snaith relating to women studied at Queen Charlotte's Maternity and Hillingdon Hospitals, and the Newcastle General Hospital, approximate figures for the likely incidence during pregnancy can be constructed (Table 6.1).

Table 6.1   Calculated frequency of endocarditis in pregnant women

Frequency of rheumatic heart disease	1:222
Frequency of mitral regurgitation (pure, or with stenosis)	1:840
Frequency of mitral regurgitation with endocarditis	1:10 000

Although all patients with valvar lesions, whether congenital or acquired, are at risk of infective endocarditis, in practice, those with rheumatic mitral regurgitation, either pure, or associated with mitral stenosis, are the most likely to develop endocarditis during pregnancy. 26·5% of the women in the series of Szekely and Snaith had mitral regurgitation, and 8·5% of these developed endocarditis during pregnancy. Endocarditis did not occur in women with other cardiac disease. All seven cases of endocarditis arising in pregnancy and the puerperium described by Mendelson had mitral incompetence. Particular attention should, therefore, be paid to prophylaxis of endocarditis in this high-risk group. Since early heart failure will arise in some 50% of women with endocarditis in pregnancy, it seems not unreasonable to propose that a full therapeutic regimen be instituted in women with mitral regurgitation, on the slightest suspicion of endocarditis and without awaiting the results of culture. We have recorded failure of what seemed adequate prophylaxis twice during pregnancy, and, now, would not hesitate to substitute a therapeutic for a prophylactic regimen if suspicion arose (Barnes and Hurley, 1963; de Swiet et al., 1975). Delay in starting therapy is thought by Mendelson to contribute to the discrepancy between recovery from infective endocarditis (60–75%) and the theoretical level of bacteriological cure (95%).

Manipulation of infected teeth is the most frequent, and the usual proximate cause of infective endocarditis, and has long been recognized (Janeway, 1899; Horder, 1909). Not all authorities (Simon and Goodwin, 1971) regard the relationship as proven. A variety of situations exist in the oral cavity

71

which, at least theoretically, may act as foci of infection and the source of distant metastases. They include infected periapical lesions such as granuloma, cyst or abscess, infected root canals, and periodontal disease especially when accompanied by manipulation or dental extraction. Investigators using an aseptic method of entrance into periapical granuloma through the root canal *in situ* have shown that, although streptococci are yielded by some, the lesions are often sterile (Sommer and Crowley, 1940; Ostrander and Crowley, 1948). For this reason, the possibility that such give rise to focal infection is thought to be minimal (Slater *et al.*, 1974). Teeth with infected root canals are potent as a source for dissemination of pathogenic bacteria although not all yield positive cultures (Morse and Yates, 1941), and bacteraemia has been found to be closely related to the severity or degree of periodontal disease after manipulation of the gingiva or, more commonly, after tooth extraction. Lewis and Grant (1923) suggested the possibility of the 'almost physiological entry' of organisms into the bloodstream of the average individual commenting that from the standpoint of pathology, the importance of defective heart valves lay in its indication of the frequency with which innocuous invasion of the blood-stream occurs amongst the general population. Okell and Elliott (1935) tested this hypothesis, and showed that within a few moments of the extraction of teeth from obviously septic mouths, a transient streptococcal bacteraemia, lasting a few minutes, occurred in 75% of cases. Even in patients with no obvious gum disease, tooth extraction was followed by transient streptococcal bacteraemia in 34% of cases. They found, also, that 10·9% of 110 persons with septic mouths, whose blood was sampled only on one occasion, had streptococcal bacteraemia, irrespective of any operative intervention. Tooth extraction, in some of these individuals, increased the colony count in the bloodstream. No close relationship could be shown between postoperative bacteraemia and pyrexia, although in 14 of 20 patients with pyorrhoea, tooth extraction was followed by elevation of the body temperature (99°F to 102°F) within 4–9 hours of operation. Mitchell and Helman (1953) have reviewed much of the literature pertaining to periodontal disease as a potential focus of infection. Observations on rocking of teeth in their sockets have shown that this favours bacteraemia (Elliot, 1939); Burket and Burn (1937) used the tracer microbe *Serratia marcescens* to demonstrate the relationship, recovering it from the bloodstream after painting it on the gingival margin before extraction.

The evidence indicates overwhelmingly that extraction of teeth, and even minor oral procedures such as cleaning and filling (Harvey and Capone, 1961), and brushing may produce transient bacteraemia, especially in persons with severe gingival disease. Organisms other than streptococci, including diphtheroids and *Staphylococcus albus*, and rarely, *Staphylococcus aureus*, also may enter the bloodstream. The risk of infective endocarditis following tooth extraction in susceptible individuals has been calculated as 1:533.

The evidence relating endocarditis to dental manipulation rests on case reports of endocarditis following tooth extraction, on the fact that the organism commonly present iş *Str. viridans* (see below) a commensal of the mouth, and on the occurrence of *Str. viridans* bacteraemia after tooth extraction. Though less attention has been paid to them, situations other than dental sepsis and manipulations within the oral cavity may occasion the entry of microbes into the bloodstream. Severe dental sepsis and caries is uncommon in children, and Zakrzewski and Keith (1965) recorded only four instances, one of caries and three of tooth extractions, in 50 children with endocarditis. They included, in their antecedent factors, a variety of conditions, including wounds, infection of a Holter valve, burns, osteomyelitis, circumcision and catheterization, recording a large number of staphylococcal infections, as well as those due to *Str. viridans*. Feinstein, Petersdorf and Browder (1961) list the most common paths of entry for micro-organisms into the bloodstream as:

(1) the mouth, gums and teeth
(2) the upper respiratory tract, particularly the tonsils and sinuses
(3) the urinary tract, in males
(4)ʻ the genital tract, in females, and
(5) direct entry

Entry following dental sepsis and manipulations on teeth has been discussed above. Other surgical procedures involving the oropharynx also result in entry of microbes into the bloodstream. Thus, Elliott (1939) and Rhoads *et al.* (1955) recorded that cultures taken immediately after tonsillectomy were positive in 30–40% of patients. Catheter fever, with entry of coliforms into the bloodstream was well known before the antibiotic era (Barrington and Wright, 1930), and bacteraemia of the order of 50–60% is a common occurrence after surgical procedures on the lower urinary tract. Endocarditis has been recorded as a complication of urethral dilatation and prostatectomy.

Far less well documented, with respect to direct studies on the incidence of bacteraemia, is the likelihood of the genital tract acting as a source of infection, particularly during parturition. Hook and Kaye (1962) state that, in common with other manipulations on grossly infected areas, dilatation and curettage of the uterus after septic abortion, as well as postpartum infection itself, constitute risks to those with valvar disease, but there seem to be only four studies assessing the incidence of transient bacteraemia, and one of these is unpublished. Redleaf and Fadell (1959) found an overall incidence of 15% positive cultures in 101 patients; 4% were positive at the end of the third stage of labour, and a further 11% were positive on the day following labour. Fourteen of the isolates were staphylococci, and one was an α-haemolytic streptococcus. Ramsey and Swartwout (1958) studied 74 cultures from 17 patients without observing a positive culture. Baker, with Hubell (1967) extended earlier observations (Baker *et al.*, 1966) by repeating a study of postpartum asymptomatic bacteraemia, sampling the blood-stream of parturient women 15 minutes, 30 minutes, 12 hours and 24 hours postpartum, and finding that 20 of 2583 blood cultures from 579 patients (0·77%) were positive. Aerobic and anaerobic Gram-negative rods, streptococci and staphylococci were isolated, and some of the patients had symptoms. The previous study had shown that 0·5% of 396 subjects had positive blood cultures without symptoms, but the later study which included specimens taken during the more critical, immediate postpartum period, demonstrated an incidence of asymptomatic puerperal bacteraemia of 1·3%. Since the incidence was so much lower than that following dental extraction, the advisability of prophylaxis during delivery was questioned. The paucity of studies dealing with entry of microbes into the bloodstream at or about labour and immediately postpartum does not betoken a disinclination on the part of physicians to account this period as one of grave risk for their patients, but rather stresses the notoriety of the risk which, formerly, often resulted in puerperal sepsis and death. The many factors that have operated to reduce the risk of septicaemia in obstetric practice must also have played a part in lessening the risk of endocarditis in susceptible patients during childbirth.

The division of endocarditis into acute and subacute forms is not exact, and it has been proposed that endocarditis be designated by the causative organism. Most authors now use the term infective endocarditis. When considering the antecedent history, the terminology of the disease becomes important. The term subacute bacterial endocarditis was sometimes reserved to those cases caused by *Str. viridans*, and in such series, it is not surprising that dental sepsis plays an important role as the source of the infection, accounting probably for 1 in 4. When all cases of infective endocarditis are considered, *Str. viridans*, though still important, is seen to account for less than half of all cases. Thus, Barber (1959) drew attention to the change in the bacterial aetiology in the post-penicillin era in patients who died. The incidence of *Str. viridans* had fallen from 61% to 35%. A *Lancet* editorial (1967) emphasized that valve infections with other more virulent and sometimes antibiotic resistant organisms are becoming increasingly troublesome in patients of all ages, although particularly so in older patients.

There are tantalizing suggestions that risk of endocarditis is greater during pregnancy and childbirth. Thus, Bramwell (1948) called attention to a high incidence in pregnant women, seven of his 22 cases occurring during pregnancy. Of Wheeler's (1960) 200 cases, nine were precipitated by abortion or delivery. Cates and Christie (1951) record three postpartum cases and one following abortion. Geraci and Martin (1954) record five out of 33 cases of enterococcal endocarditis associated with delivery, abortion or dilatation and curettage. The study of Pedowitz and Hellman (1953) did not show that pregnancy itself was associated with an unusually high risk of relapse in women with healed endocarditis (9·4%), although three of eight women who relapsed did so during the puerperium, and none of these had had prophylactic antibiotics. Their study dispelled the notion that endocarditis is a rare complication of pregnancy, since the writers reported 35 cases occurring during pregnancy, a greater number than that reported in the preceding world literature from 1941. It is probable that the incidence of postpartum endocarditis would relate directly to the aseptic and antiseptic measures taken during delivery, and that its incidence would vary accordingly. It does not seem to have been a common disease in the obstetric practice of Queen Charlotte's Hospital before the antibiotic era (Table 6.2). Over the relevant

Table 6.2   Endocarditis in pregnancy: QCMH

	No. of cardiac cases	Endocarditis
1910–1914	78	1
1922–1926	95	1
1932–1936	113	1
Total	286	3

period, there were many cases of severe, often fatal puerperal infections (18 in the 5 years 1910–1914). In one of these cases, endocarditis caused by *B. coli (Escherichia coli)* seems to have followed pyelitis, and occurred at the 30th week, emphasizing that sources other than the teeth, and microbes other than *Str. viridans*, may be implicated in endocarditis in obstetric practice.

Modern taxonomical methods allow more exact identification of microbes, so that there is hope that the pathogenesis of common serious infectious disease may be further elucidated. *Str. viridans* is no longer deemed a sufficiently exact designation in epidemiological work, and the streptococci isolated from patients with endocarditis are predominantly, but not exclusively, *Str. sanguis, Str. mitior*, and *Str. mutans* (Parker and Ball, 1976). The vagina abounds with streptococci, but few have been identified with this degree of precision (de Louvois *et al.*, 1975).

The prevention of endocarditis begins with the prevention and treatment of infection by the Lancefield A streptococcus, which is generally accepted as playing a causative role in rheumatic fever. While endocarditis may occur in previously undamaged hearts, and in congenitally malformed hearts, those damaged by rheumatic carditis are most frequently affected. The incidence of Group A streptococcal disease is falling in western communities (Tables 6.3 and 6.4), and, so too, is the incidence of rheumatic fever. *Str. pyogenes* (Lancefield Group A) was isolated, formerly, from about 70% of those who died of puerperal sepsis, but its isolation is now a great rarity in obstetric practice. Despite the greatly lessened risk of streptococcal infection, and, thus, of recurrence of rheumatic fever exacerbating, or producing rheumatic carditis, continuous prophylaxis is still used widely in susceptible patients. Monthly injections of benzathine penicillin are used by some, and others favour daily, oral penicillin. In addition, treatment of established streptococcal infection should be early and adequate. Erythromycin has

Table 6.3   Deaths from scarlet fever, England and Wales, per million population, 1871–1950*

1871–1880	720
1881–1890	340
1891–1900	160
1901–1910	110
1911–1920	46
1921–1930	23
1931–1940	11
1950	0·7

* Data compiled by Paul, H., 1964

been used in those allergic to penicillin. Evaluation of these regimes of prophylaxis is not straightforward. Patients on long-term penicillin harbour resistant streptococci and this may be important (Garrod and Waterworth, 1962) if they are exposed to a situation where there is risk that endocarditis may supervene.

Table 6.4   Queen Charlotte's Maternity Hospital reports 1932–1968. Deaths from puerperal sepsis

Mortality rates expressed as percentages	
1932	11·2
1935*	11·1
1937	4·9
1938	3·9
1947	Nil
1968	0·8†

* Prontosil used January, 1936
† *Cl. welchii*

The goals of prophylaxis of endocarditis are: to reduce the magnitude and duration of bacteraemia and to eradicate bacteria implanted on the endocardium. It is dangerous to attempt sterilization of a likely source site, since this may selectively encourage the emergence of resistant strains. Many drugs have been used either alone, or in combination, and most are directed against *Str. viridans*, the most notorious of the causative agents. They have comprised tetracycline, crystalline procaine penicillin, alone or in combination with streptomycin, cephaloridine or cephalexin, ampicillin or cephazolin with gentamicin, methecillin. Szekely and Snaith favour crystalline penicillin or ampicillin and/or cephaloridine or cephalexin, and Mendelson favours penicillin and streptomycin over the period of labour. Durack (1975) recommends ampicillin and gentamicin for operations on the urinary tract, and, in view of our failure with cephaloridine, this is the regimen currently favoured at Queen Charlotte's Hospital during labour. It is probably important that prophylaxis over the period of labour should not be with those drugs that have been used for continuous prophylaxis of rheumatic fever.

A *Lancet* editorial (1976) states that antibiotic prophylaxis should be used as long as its efficacy remains reasonably credible. The basis of credibility lies in knowledge of the *in vitro* activity of certain antibiotics, notably penicillin, against the microbes that frequently cause endocarditis, for example, *Str. viridans*; in belief that a bactericidal agent should be used, since the deposition of bacteria on the valves though probably mechanical would leave the microbes free to multiply once a bacteristatic agent had been withdrawn; in use of short-term treatment, in the hope that microbes reaching the valves will not include 'persisters', and, finally, on experimental observations. The latter confirm the protective powers of penicillin and streptomycin, vancomycin, phenoxymethyl penicillin, and mixtures of benzyl penicillin with a long-acting penicillin. We are urged to remember that some people are sensitive to penicillin, and some bacteria are not. Ampicillin has proved a useful drug in the treatment of incipient puerperal sepsis, and, combined with gentamicin, should give reasonably broad, safe and bactericidal prophylaxis during parturition.

References

Baker, T. H. and Hubell, R. (1967). Reappraisal of asymptomatic puerperal bacteraemia. *Am. J. Obstet. Gynecol.*, **97**, 575

Baker, T. H., Machikawa, J. H. and Stapleton, J. J. (1966). Asymptomatic puerperal bacteraemia. *Am. J. Obstet. Gynecol.*, **94**, 903

Barber, Mary (1959). Bacterial endocarditis. *Proc. R. Soc. Med.*, **53**, 554

Barnes, C. G. (1970). *Medical Disorders in Obstetric Practice*, 3rd Ed. (Oxford: Blackwell Scientific Publications)

Barnes, C. G. and Hurley, Rosalinde (1963). Antibiotic cover for dental extractions. *Br. Med. J.*, **2**, 1205

Barrington, F. J. F. and Wright, H. D. (1930). Bacteraemia following operations on the urethra. *J. Pathol. Bacteriol.*, **33**, 871

Bramwell, C. (1948). Subacute bacterial endocarditis. *Lancet*, **ii**, 481

Burket, L. W. and Burn, C. G. (1937). Bacteremias following dental extraction: demonstration of source of bacteria by means of a non-pathogen (*Serratia marcescens*). *J. Dental Res.*, **16**, 521

Burwell, C. S. and Metcalfe, J. (1958). *Heart Disease and Pregnancy: Physiology and Management.* (Boston, Mass: Little Brown and Co.)

Campbell, M. (1968). The incidence and later distribution of malformations of the heart. In H. Watson (ed.) *Paediatric Cardiology.* (London: Lloyd-Luke)

Campbell, M. (1973). Incidence of cardiac malformations at birth and later, and neonatal mortality. *Br. Heart J.*, **35**, 189

Cates, J. E. and Christie, R. V. (1951). Subacute treated endocarditis — a review of 442 patients treated in 14 centres. *Q. J. Med.*, **2**, 93

Clarkson, P. M. and Barrett-Boyes, B. G. (1970). Bacterial endocarditis following homograft replacement of the aortic valve. *Circulation*, **42**, 987

Copeland, W. E., Wooley, C. F., Ryan, J. M., Runco, V. and Levin, H. S. (1963). Pregnancy and congenital heart disease. *Am. J. Obstet. Gynecol.*, **86**, 107

Durack, D. T. (1975). Current practice in prevention of bacterial endocarditis. *Br. Heart J.*, **37**, 478

Editorial (1967). Bacterial endocarditis: a changing pattern. *Lancet*, **i**, 605

Editorial (1976). Prophylaxis of bacterial endocarditis. Faith, hope and charitable interpretations. *Lancet*, **i**, 519

Edwards, J. E. (1973). Bacterial endocarditis and prosthetic valves. *Circulation*, **47**, 987

Elliott, S. D. (1939). Bacteraemia following tonsillectomy. *Lancet*, **ii**, 589

Elliott, S. D. (1939). Bacteraemia and oral sepsis. *Proc. R. Soc. Med.*, **32**, 747

Feinstein, A. R., Petersdorf, R. G. and Browder, Ann. (1961). Prophylaxis of poststreptococcal sequelae and bacterial endocarditis. *J. Pediatr.*, **58**, 164

Garrod, L. P. and Waterworth, Pamela M. (1962). The risks of dental extraction during penicillin treatment. *Br. Heart J.*, **24**, 39

Geraci, J. E. and Martin, V. J. (1954). Antibiotic therapy of bacterial endocarditis: Subacute enterococcal endocarditis: clinical, pathologic, and therapeutic considerations of 33 cases. *Circulation*, **10**, 173

Hamilton, B. E. (1947). Report from the cardiac clinic of the Boston Lying-In Hospital for the first twenty-five years. *Am. Heart J.*, **33**, 663

Harvey, W. P. and Capone, M. A. (1961). Bacterial endocarditis related to cleaning and filling of teeth. *Am. J. Cardiol.*, **7**, 793

Hayward, G. (1960). Bacterial endocarditis. *Proc. R. Soc. Med.*, **53**, 551

Hook, E. W. and Kaye, D. (1962). Prophylaxis of bacterial endocarditis. *J. Chron. Dis.*, **15**, 635

Horder, T. J. (1909). Infective endocarditis: Analysis of 150 cases and with special reference to the chronic form of the disease. *Q. J. Med.*, **2**, 289

Hurley, Rosalinde (1972). Penicillin treatment in obstetrics and gynaecology. *J. R. Coll. Physicians, London*, **6**, 151

Janeway, E. G. (1899). Certain clinical observations upon heart disease. *Med. News*, **75**, 257

Keith, J. D., Rowe, R. D. and Vlad, P. (1967). *Heart Disease in Infancy and Childhood*, 2nd Ed. (Toronto: Macmillan)

Lewis, T. and Grant, R. T. (1923). Observation relating to subacute endocarditis. *Heart*, **10**, 21

de Louvois, J., Hurley, Rosalinde and Stanley, Valerie C. (1975). Microbial flora of the genital tract during pregnancy: Relationship to morbidity. *J. Clin. Pathol.*, **28**, 731

Mendelson, C. L. (1960). *Cardiac Disease in Pregnancy*. (Philadelphia: F. A. Davis)

Mitchell, D. F. and Helman, E. Z. (1953). The role of periodontal foci of infection in systemic disease: an evaluation of the literature. *J. Am. Dent. Assoc.*, **46**, 32

Morse, F. W., Jr. and Yates, M. F. (1941). Follow-up studies of root filled teeth in relation to bacteriologic findings. *J. Am. Dent. Assoc.*, **28**, 956

Okell, C. C. and Elliott, S. D. (1935). Bacteraemia and oral sepsis. *Lancet*, **ii**, 869

Ostrander, F. D. and Crowley, M. C. (1948). The effectiveness of clinical treatment of pulp involved teeth as determined by bacteriological methods. *J. Endodont.*, **3**, 6

Parker, M. T. and Ball, Lyn C. (1976). Streptococci and aerococci associated with systemic infection in man. *J. Med. Microbiol.*, **9**, 276

Pedowitz, P. and Hellman, L. (1953). Pregnancy and healed bacterial endocarditis. *Am. J. Obstet. Gynecol.*, **66**, 294

Ramsey, L. and Swartwout, J., cited by Burwell, C. S. and Metcalfe, J. (1958). *Heart Disease and Pregnancy: Physiology and Management*. (Boston, Mass: Little, Brown and Co.)

Redleaf, P. D. and Fadell, E. J. (1959). Bacteremia during parturition; prevention of subacute bacterial endocarditis. *J. Am. Med. Assoc.*, **169**, 1284

Rhoads, P. S., Sibley, J. R. and Billings, C. E. (1955). Bacteremia following tonsillectomy. Effect of preoperative bacteremia and bacterial content of tonsils. *J. Am. Med. Assoc.*, **157**, 877

Simon, D. S. and Goodwin, J. F. (1971). Should good teeth be extracted to prevent *Str. viridans* endocarditis? *Lancet*, i, 1207

Slater, W. G., Hine, K. and Levy, B. M. (1974). *A Textbook of Oral Pathology*, 3rd Ed. (New York: W. B. Saunders)

Sommer, R. F. and Crowley, M. C. (1940). Bacteriologic verification of roentgenographic findings in pulp involved teeth. *J. Am. Dent. Assoc.*, **27**, 723

de Swiet, M., de Louvois, J. and Hurley, Rosalinde (1975). Failure of cephalosporins to prevent bacterial endocarditis during labour. *Lancet*, ii, 257

Szekely, P. and Snaith, L. (1974). *Heart Disease and Pregnancy*. (Edinburgh and London: Churchill Livingstone)

Wheeler, C. H. (1960). Personal communication to Mendelson

Wilson, May G. (1940–1961). *Advances in Rheumatic Fever*. Hoeber Medical Division (New York: Harper and Row)

Zakrzewski, T. and Keith, J. D. (1965). Bacterial endocarditis in infants and children. *J. Pediatr.*, **67**, 1179

Discussion

Herxheimer, A., London: Professor Hurley, do you reserve antibiotic prophylaxis for patients with mitral incompetences?

Hurley: No we do not.

Herxheimer: If not, why not?

Hurley: I agree this would be a logical practice but we do not, because there is a theoretical risk of bacterial endocarditis with all valve lesions. I do not think we are justified in reserving our prophylaxis to mitral incompetence just because in the published theories the lesion has been confined to this region.

Herxheimer: But surely you are trying to counter a real rather than a theoretical risk.

Hurley: I take your point but I must admit that we are responding largely to a theoretical risk.

7
Drug Treatment and Prophylaxis of Thromboembolism in Pregnancy

M. de SWIET, ELIZABETH LETSKY and HEATHER J. MELLOWS

INTRODUCTION

The Confidential Enquiry into Maternal Mortality reveals that in the years 1970–72 in England and Wales 61 of 355 maternal deaths (17%) were due to pulmonary embolism. Pulmonary embolism has remained second to abortion as the most common cause of maternal death in England and Wales since 1958. Approximately one-third of deaths occurred in the antenatal period, and two-thirds, *post-partum*. An increasing tendency towards antenatal thromboembolism rather than postnatal thromboembolism has also been noted by Henderson and his colleagues (1972). Predisposing factors to thromboembolism in pregnancy (DHSS, 1975) are age, obesity, Caesarean section and other operative forms of delivery, oestrogen treatment to suppress lactation (DHSS, 1975; Daniel *et al.*, 1967), and also possibly the presence of HbS either as sickle cell disease or sickle cell trait (DHSS, 1975). Changing patterns of obstetric practice and the awareness of the predisposing causes of thromboembolism may account for the increased proportion of antenatal thromboembolism. For example, obstetricians are aware of the risk of oestrogen treatment and therefore do not advise it in the puerperium particularly after Caesarean section. In contrast, more patients are admitted antenatally, often for long periods of bed-rest and this may account for some of the increase in *ante-partum* thromboembolism.

It is widely believed that an episode of previous thromboembolism predisposes patients to thromboembolism in pregnancy. Some believe the risk

81

to be especially high if the original episode of thromboembolism occurred while the patient was taking the contraceptive pill or during pregnancy. Yet there is little epidemiological data concerning these interrelationships. Vessey (1974) re-examined the pregnancy experience of 42 patients who had originally had thromboembolism whilst taking the contraceptive pill. He compared them with 42 controls who had thromboembolism unassociated with the pill. There were 24 pregnancies in each group and in each group there were three episodes of thromboembolism in pregnancy. The risk of thromboembolism in pregnancy in a patient who has previously had an episode of thromboembolism therefore appears to be approximately 12% whether or not the original episode occurred whilst the patient was on the pill. In contrast, the risk of thromboembolism at times other than pregnancy was much greater in the non-pill than the pill group.

Because of the 12% risk of repeat thromboembolism, which is such a potent cause of maternal mortality, we therefore decided to give prophylactic anticoagulants to all women in pregnancy who had had a previous well-documented episode of thromboembolism. We used a standardized anticoagulant regime and have presented our results in all patients including those requiring therapeutic as well as prophylactic anticoagulants.

AN OPEN STUDY OF ANTICOAGULANT TREATMENT IN PREGNANCY

Subjects

Anticoagulants have been used in 27 patients at Queen Charlotte's Maternity Hospital between 1975 and 1976. During this period there were approximately 6400 deliveries. The indications for anticoagulant treatment are

Table 7.1 Indications for anticoagulant treatment in pregnancy and the peurperium

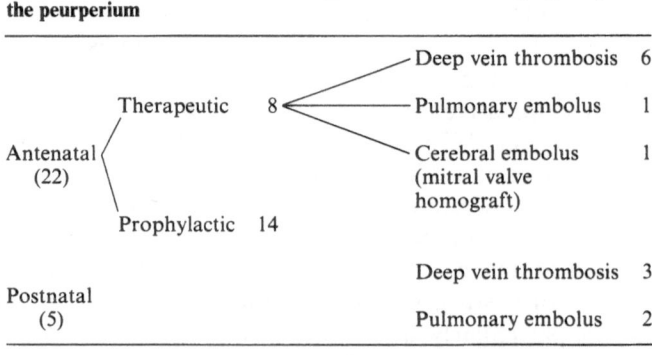

given in Table 7.1. The prophylactic group includes two patients who required anticoagulants for artificial heart valves as well as 12 patients who were given anticoagulants because of previous thromboembolism.

Anticoagulant technique

The two patients with artificial heart valves were already taking warfarin when they became pregnant. Of the 12 patients who took anticoagulants because of previous thromboembolism, 11 started warfarin after 14 weeks' gestation. This delay occurred partly because of the risk of warfarin tera-togenicity (Kerber, 1968) and partly because the patients presented relatively late in pregnancy. One patient presented early in pregnancy having had a recent deep vein thrombosis and was treated with subcutaneous heparin (see below) from the 6th to the 14th week of pregnancy. The eight patients with thromboembolism in pregnancy all presented after 14 weeks' gestation. Our overall plan was to continue warfarin controlled by prothrombin time until 36 weeks' gestation. At that time, because of the risk of fetal bleeding (Villasanta, 1965), the patients were admitted to hospital and given sub-cutaneous heparin, 10000° b.d. Heparin assays were performed in all patients (Denson and Bonnar, 1973). Twelve of the 22 patients treated antenatally were able to give themselves subcutaneous heparin and were discharged from hospital. Subcutaneous heparin was continued through labour and for 72 hours after delivery. 24 hours after delivery, patients restarted warfarin. This was continued for 3 weeks in the group that were given anticoagulants because of previous thromboembolism, indefinitely in the patients with artificial heart valves and for at least 6 weeks in the 12 patients who were given anticoagulants because of thromboembolism in this pregnancy.

The 12 patients that presented with thromboembolism in this pregnancy were treated in addition with therapeutic levels of heparin 10000° i.v., 6-hourly for 48 hours until they achieved anticoagulant levels of warfarin. No patients presented with thromboembolism between 36 weeks' gestation and delivery. If they had done so, our plan was to treat them with therapeutic levels of heparin (10000° i.v., 6-hourly) for 1 week and then reduce heparin treatment to the subcutaneous regime.

The outcome of anticoagulant treatment

The infant

There were 23 infants delivered from the 22 mothers who took anticoagulants antenatally including one set of twins. There was one neonatal death associ-ated with premature labour at 29 weeks' gestation. All the remaining 22 infants appeared normal with no evidence of congenital abnormalities. One infant had a cephalhaematoma associated with a normal delivery and one infant had bruising associated with a rotation and delivery by Kielland's forceps, but in neither of these cases was the bleeding any greater than might be expected from the degree of trauma associated with the delivery.

The mother

There was no significant bleeding in the antenatal period except that two patients developed haematuria. In one patient this was transient and no problem but in the other patient who started bleeding at 25 weeks' gestation, anticoagulant treatment was very difficult to control; the prothrombin time bore little relationship to the quality of warfarin that she was supposed to be taking. We therefore did not believe that she could safely be anticoagulated with warfarin and she was admitted to hospital and treated with sub-cutaneous heparin.

Table 7.2   Methods of delivery in patients on anticoagulants (22)

Caesarian section	3	Spontaneous vaginal delivery	10
Vaginal deliveries	19	Forceps and Ventouse	8
		Breech	1
Episiotomy	14		
1° tear	3		
2° tear	2		

Labour was in general uneventful in these patients and the incidence of instrumental delivery showed the same pattern as in the rest of the hospital population (see Table 7.2). There was a rather higher incidence of perineal tears than we would normally find in our hospital population, probably due to a reluctance on the part of some attendants to perform an episiotomy in patients taking anticoagulants. Patients taking anticoagulants were not given epidural anaesthetics because of the risk of haemorrhage into the epidural space.

Seven of the 22 (32%) patients who had been taking anticoagulants before delivery had *post-partum* haemorrhages estimated to be greater than 500 ml. However, three of the *post-partum* haemorrhages were probably due to obstetric intervention rather than to anticoagulant treatment. In one patient the cervix was cut; another patient required a large episiotomy for Ventouse delivery of a 4·5 kg infant and the third patient required a manual removal of retained placenta.

Four of the 22 patients who had been taking anticoagulants antenatally (18%) did have *post-partum* haemorrhages requiring transfusion between 1 and 7 litres, which could, in part, be ascribed to anticoagulant treatment.

One patient, who was very obese and was taking prophylactic anticoagulants because of a previous deep vein thrombosis, bled from the abdominal wound of a Caesarian section whilst she was receiving subcutaneous heparin 10 000° b.d., 24 hours after delivery. Three patients bled from the genital tract between 7 and 11 days after delivery when they were taking warfarin. In none of these cases was the prothrombin time outside the therapeutic range. Each had scanty retained products of conception when the uterus was evacuated but it is difficult to believe that the retained products were the sole cause of *post-partum* haemorrhage in these patients.

None of the five patients who were anticoagulated *post-partum* because of thromboembolism in the pueperium had any bleeding problems. There was no case of thromboembolism in any of the patients who were being anticoagulated. However, one of the patients, anticoagulated because of an artificial heart vaɩve, had a massive *post-partum* haemorrhage. Anticoagulant therapy was stopped and she suffered two cerebral emboli.

Lactation

Twelve of the mothers who took anticoagulants before and after delivery were breast feeding when they were discharged from hospital. There were no bleeding complications in the infants. There was no warfarin detectable in the breast milk of six mothers nor in their infants' blood (Baty *et al.*, 1976). These infants all had prothrombin times which were normal for their ages.

DISCUSSION

We found that the risk of *post-partum* haemorrhage in patients who were anticoagulated at delivery varied between 18% and 32% depending on whether the bleeding was thought to be due to obstetric manoeuvres or anticoagulant therapy. Although severaɩ authors (Hirsch *et al.*, 1970; Finnerty and MacKay, 1962; Taylor, 1965; Quenneville *et al.*, 1959; Pridmore *et al.*, 1975) have found no increased risk of maternal bleeding due to anticoagulants, Henderson *et al.* (1972) found that amongst the 15 of 17 patients anticoagulated who had some degree of morbidity, two had *post-partum* haemorrhages. Ramsey (1975) reported one case of *post-partum* haemorrhage due to heparin therapy despite 'careful' control of the clotting time and Mueller and Lebherz (1969) found that three of 10 patients anti-coagulated with heparin had *post-partum* haemorrhages. The quantity of heparin given to our patients, 10000° subcutaneously b.d. is not sufficient to affect the whole blood clotting time in pregnancy. Isolated heparin assays performed in every patient showed that the heparin level was consistently less than 0·1 units per ml. Bonnar reports that only heparin levels in excess of 0·6 units/ml are associated with bleeding (Bonnar, 1975). We did not repeatedly assay heparin levels in our patients.

Furthermore, three of the four patients whose *post-partum* haemorrhages were thought to be due to anticoagulants, bled while they were taking warfarin. We suggest that patients are more likely to bleed while they are taking warfarin than when they are given small quantities of heparin. Very

85

small doses of heparin inhibit the activation of factor X, and this does not affect the whole blood clotting time. In contrast, warfarin interferes with the hepatic synthesis of several factors and does prolong coagulation. As a result of this study we intend to delay the introduction of warfarin treatment in the pueperium until 8–10 days *post-partum*. Subcutaneous heparin will be continued until patients are established on warfarin treatment. Because of the risk of *post-partum* haemorrhage in patients taking warfarin, we also intend to perform an ultrasound examination of the uterus before commencing warfarin therapy. In these patients evacuation of the uterus will be advised if there are retained products even in the absence of significant bleeding. It is our impression that many patients have asymptomatic retained products of conception, but these are more likely to cause bleeding in the presence of warfarin therapy.

In our series, the 23 babies delivered from mothers who had received warfarin antenatally appeared normal. Nevertheless, the problem of warfarin teratogenicity remains unsolved. Tejani (1973) questioned Kerber's (1968) and Di Saia's (1966) original observations that warfarin causes nasal hypoplasia, optic atrophy, and mental retardation, because Kerber's patient had taken other drugs and Di Saia's patient had positive serology for syphilis. However, further reports of the same syndrome have appeared (Becker *et al.*, 1975; Shaul *et al.*, 1975; Pettifor and Benson, 1975) and Holzgreve *et al.* (1976) has recently reviewed the literature and found reports of 16 abnormal children born after anticoagulant treatment. He postulates that anticoagulants taken early in pregnancy may cause nasal hypoplasia and stippled epiphyses whereas anticoagulants taken late in pregnancy may cause optic atrophy and microcephaly even if there is no overt fetal bleeding. These defects arising later in pregnancy may not be apparent at birth. We are therefore making yearly examinations of all babies born to mothers taking anticoagulants. It would appear to be prudent to recommend mothers to avoid taking oral anticoagulants in early pregnancy. Those patients who develop thromboembolism, or who need prophylaxis in the first trimester, should be offered subcutaneous heparin until 13 weeks' gestation. The patients who are taking anticoagulants for artificial heart valves before they become pregnant are most at risk. It is likely that the risk of early teratogenicity due to anticoagulants is low since the total number of affected children reported is small. Nevertheless, patients with artificial heart valves who are contemplating pregnancy should be informed of this risk and advised of the alternative method of anticoagulation available (subcutaneous heparin).

We will not know whether the apparently high incidence of microcephaly and optic atrophy is a real effect of anticoagulants, until further long-term studies are available of the infants of *all* women in a series who have received oral anticoagulants in pregnancy. At present, only isolated reports of cases are available and these may reflect selection bias.

We found no contra-indication to mothers breast feeding their infants while taking warfarin. Pridmore *et al.* (1975) found that such infants did not have prolonged prothrombin times. We confirmed this in our study and also could find no evidence that warfarin was present in the infants' blood or mothers' milk (Baty *et al.*, 1976). However, it is quite possible that phenindione, the other widely used oral anticoagulant is secreted in breast milk because of the report (Eckstein and Jack, 1970) of bleeding in a breast fed infant whose mother took the drug.

In summary, there seems little doubt that anticoagulant treatment is indicated in patients who have thromboembolism in pregnancy, since the maternal mortality untreated is about 15% (Villasanta, 1965). Similarly, patients with artificial heart valves should continue to take anticoagulant therapy. Three of 11 patients who did not, suffered cerebral emboli (Tejani, 1973). There is still uncertainty whether patients who have had thromboembolism in the past should be given prophylactic anticoagulants in pregnancy, and, if so, by what regime. Only further studies will show whether the 12% risk of repeat thromboembolism is greater than the risk of *postpartum* haemorrhage and possible risk of late fetal malformation.

Acknowledgements

It is a pleasure to acknowledge the help of our obstetric colleagues at Queen Charlotte's Maternity Hospital who generously referred patients to us. We are also grateful to Susan Cowley for preparing the manuscript.

References

Badaracco, M. A. and Vessey, M. (1974). Recurrence of venous thromboembolic disease and use of oral contraceptives. *Br. Med. J.*, **1**, 215

Baty, J. D., Breckenbridge, A., Lewis, P. J., Orme, M., Serlin, M. J. and Sibeon, R. G. (1976). May mothers taking warfarin breast feed their infants? *Br. J. Clin. Pharmacol.*, **3**, 969

Becker, M. H., Genieser, N. B., Feingold, M. *et al.* (1975). Chondrodysplasia punctata: is maternal warfarin therapy a factor? *Am. J. Dis. Child.*, **129**, 356

Bonnar, J. (1975). Thromboembolism in obstetric and gynaecological patients. In A. N. Nicolaides (ed.) *Thromboembolism. Aetiology, Advances in Prevention and Management.* p. 324. (Lancaster: MTP Press Limited)

Daniel, D. G., Campbell, H. and Turnbull, A. C. (1967). Puerperal thrombo-embolism and suppression of lactation. *Lancet*, **ii**, 287

Denson, K. W. E. and Bonnar, J. (1973). The measurement of heparin: a method based on the potentiation of anti-factor X a. *Thromb. Diath. Haemorrh.*, **30**, 471

Department of Health and Social Security (1975). *Report on Confidential Enquiries into Maternal Deaths in England and Wales 1970–1972*, p. 140. (London: Her Majesty's Stationery Office)

Di Saia, P. J. (1966). Pregnancy and delivery of a patient with a mitral valve prosthesis. *Obstet. Gynecol.*, **28**, 469

Eckstein, H. and Jack, B. (1970). Breast feeding and anticoagulant therapy. *Lancet*, **i**, 672

Finnerty, J. J. and MacKay, B. R. (1962). Antepartum thrombophlebitis and pulmonary embolism. *Obstet. Gynecol.*, **19**, 405

Henderson, S. R., Lund, C. J. and Creasman, W. T. (1972). Antepartum pulmonary embolism. *Am. J. Obstet. Gynecol.*, **112**, 476

Hirsch, J., Cade, J. F. and O'Sullivan, E. F. (1970). Clinical experience with anticoagulant therapy during pregnancy. *Br. Med. J.*, **1**, 270

Holzgreve, W., Carey, J. C. and Hall, B. D. (1976). Warfarin-induced fetal abnormalities. *Lancet*, **ii**, 914

Kerber, I. J. (1968). Pregnancy in a patient with a prosthetic mitral valve associated with a fetal abnormality attributed to warfarin sodium. *J. Am. Med. Assoc.*, **203**, 223

Mueller, M. J. and Lebherz, T. B. (1969). Antepartum thrombophlebitis. *Obstet. Gynecol.*, **34**, 874

Pettifor, J. M. and Benson, R. (1975). Congenital malformations associated with the administration of oral anticoagulants during pregnancy. *J. Paediatr.*, **86**, 459

Pridmore, B. R., Murray, K. H. and McAllen, P. M. (1975). The management of anticoagulant therapy during and after pregnancy. *Br. J. Obstet. Gynaecol.*, **82**, 740

Quenneville, G., Barton, B., McDevitt, E. and Wright, I. S. (1959). The use of anticoagulants for thrombophlebitis during pregnancy. *Am. J. Obstet. Gynecol.*, **77**, 1135

Ramsey, D. M. (1975). Thromboembolism in pregnancy. *Obstet. Gynecol.*, **45**, 129

Shaul, W. L., Emery, H. and Hall, J. G. (1975). Chondrodysplasia punctata and maternal warfarin use during pregnancy. *Am. J. Dis. Child.*, **129**, 360

Taylor, J. J. (1965). Antepartum thromboembolism. *Postgrad. Med. J.*, **41**, 80

Tejani, N. (1973). Anticoagulant therapy with cardiac valve prosthesis during pregnancy. *Obstet. Gynecol.*, **42**, 785

Villasanta, U. (1965). Thromboembolic disease in pregnancy. *Am. J. Obstet. Gynecol.*, **93**, 142

Discussion

Dargie, H. J., London: I am a little confused about Dr de Swiet's use of heparin. Surely the use of 10 000 units of heparin subcutaneously is a prophylactic regimen. Was this regimen used for the treatment of patients?

de Swiet: It was purely coincidental that none of our patients had proven thrombo-embolism after the 35th week of pregnancy. In all cases the initial incident occurred earlier in pregnancy. At this time therefore we were using prophylactic heparin. In any event recurrent thromboembolism was not a problem in the study.

Redman, C. W. G., Oxford: It has been suggested that in the use of subcutaneous heparin there is a place for screening patients for their response to these doses, before treatment is commenced. Have you thought of doing this?

de Swiet: We have thought of doing this but have not done so yet.

Dollery, C. T.: Did you control your heparin therapy in any way or did you use a fixed dose?

de Swiet: We measured heparin levels throughout but we did not have to adjust our dosage in any patient as a result of these measurements.

Stewart, C. M., London: I should like to ask Dr de Swiet about the primary post-partum haemorrhages in his series. Were these cases related to perineal damage?

de Swiet: No, the primary post-partum haemorrhages were not in any of the people who had perineal tears. They all occurred in patients who had had episiotomies.

Part 3
Medical Disorders

8
Thyroid Therapy in Pregnancy

I. D. RAMSAY

INTRODUCTION

The normal human thyroid is not palpable except in very thin individuals. Careful palpation of the neck however reveals an enlarged thyroid in up to 70% of pregnant women (Crooks *et al.*, 1964). Hyperthyroidism is diagnosed in two women out of every 1000 each year (Logan and Cushion, 1958). Since the mean age at which hyperthyroidism develops is close to that of the menopause one can assume that half of these women will be of childbearing age and in fact it has been shown that the prevalence of hyperthyroidism in pregnancy is just below one per 1000 (Javert, 1940; Kibel, 1944). Hypothyroidism seems to be slightly less common than hyperthyroidism in the community (Tunbridge *et al.*, 1976). No figures are available for its prevalence in pregnant women but in my clinic I see 50% more pregnant women with hyperthyroidism than I see with hypothyroidism.

MATERNAL THYROID PHYSIOLOGY

During pregnancy the renal clearance of iodide doubles and the plasma inorganic iodine falls; the thyroidal clearance of iodine goes up to three times the normal (Crooks *et al.*, 1964) and thyroidal ^{132}I uptakes become elevated though this investigation should not be carried out! These changes in iodine metabolism are probably responsible for the goitre formation. However, the possibility that chorionic or molar thyrotrophin (Tunbridge and Hall, 1975) may play some part in goitre formation has not been resolved.

During pregnancy the increased production of oestrogens causes the main carrier protein, thyroxine-binding globulin (TBG), to double in concentration by the end of the first trimester and it remains elevated until delivery,

93

after which it falls slowly to normal values by about 8–10 weeks post-partum. Because of the rise in TBG the number of binding sites for thyroid hormones is increased and so the total thyroxine (T_4) in the blood is greater than in the normal subject. However, not all the binding sites are saturated; indeed a lot are vacant. The triiodothyronine resin uptake (T_3RU) test can measure these vacant sites and in pregnancy will give a value which is usually in the hypothyroid range. However, the raised total T_4 and the hypothyroid T_3RU can be combined mathematically in order to give an indication of the amount of thyroxine which is circulating in the blood in the unbound state. This is called the free thyroxine index (FT_4I). Thus, in a euthyroid pregnant woman the FT_4I will fall in the normal range (Goolden et al., 1967) and it is the best indication of thyroid function in pregnancy.

The other thyroid hormone triiodothyronine (T_3) is much less readily bound to carrier proteins and only about 20% of euthyroid pregnant women have T_3s above the normal range at term (Ramsay et al., 1976). From the T_3 and the T_3RU a free triiodothyronine index (FT_3I) can be calculated. This also is in the normal range in euthyroid pregnant women (Ramsay et al., 1976).

FETAL THYROID PHYSIOLOGY

By the 12th week of gestation the fetal thyroid takes up iodine and secretes hormones. Thyroid stimulating hormone (TSH) is detectable in the blood at 78 days' of gestation and reaches a plateau concentration, maintained until term, at 16 weeks (Greenberg et al., 1970). The cord blood total T_4 is the same as that of the mother at term (Lieblich and Utiger, 1973), but I find that the cord FT_4I tends to be a little higher than that of the mother because of the lower concentrations of TBG in the fetus (Ramsay et al., 1976). Cord T_3 concentration is considerably less than in the mother, about $\frac{1}{3}$ of the value, and the same applies to FT_3I (Ramsay et al., 1976; Greenberg et al., 1970; Montalvo et al., 1973). Part of the discrepancy is made up by the presence in cord blood of an inactive form of T_3 called reverse T_3 (Chopra et al., 1975).

Cord TSH is higher than in normal adults or in the mother at term (Lieblich and Utiger, 1973; Fisher and Odell, 1969). Immediately after birth the concentration of TSH in fetal blood rises briskly and causes a peak concentration of T_4 between 24 and 48 hours (Erenberg et al., 1974). The T_4 concentration gradually falls back over the first month to that of a normal adult (Montalvo et al., 1973).

PLACENTAL TRANSFER OF HORMONES

Thyroid stimulating hormone is believed not to cross the placenta. Animal studies suggest that thyroid hormones do not cross the placenta (Erenberg *et al.*, 1974), but there is evidence in humans that a very slow transfer takes place (Grumbach and Werner, 1956; Dussault *et al.*, 1969). In a study of 29 pregnant women without thyroid disease we have found that there are significant correlations between maternal and cord FT_4I and between maternal and cord FT_3I, suggesting that transfer of both hormones takes place (Ramsay *et al.*, 1976). It could be argued that these positive correlations exist because both mother and fetus are exposed to the same environmental influences. However, the babies of mothers given thyroxine during pregnancy for either hypothyroidism or for the treatment of multinodular goitre had a higher mean FT_4I than the control babies and their TSH concentrations were significantly lower, suggesting that they had been suppressed by the T_4. This is evidence in favour of placental transfer of T_4.

HYPERTHYROIDISM IN PREGNANCY

Since hyperthyroidism tends to give rise to oligomenorrhoea or to amenorrhoea these women are usually infertile (Astwood, 1951), though pregnancies can occur in women with a mild form of the disease. Most of the patients one has to manage are already on treatment for hyperthyroidism when they become pregnant. Some of the patients become hyperthyroid while they are pregnant, though this is uncommon. The clinical diagnosis can be difficult because many of the features of hyperthyroidism may be found in normal pregnancy, such as emotional lability, heat intolerance, tachycardia, a hyperdynamic circulation and a goitre. However, there are a few pointers towards the diagnosis of hyperthyroidism. The patient may have failed to gain weight despite a good appetite, there may be a rapid sleeping pulse, she may have exophthalmos, lid lag and lid retraction and there may be a bruit over the thyroid. The best test is to take blood for T_4 and T_3RU and to calculate the FT_4I which will be raised if the patient has hyperthyroidism.

TREATMENT OF HYPERTHYROIDISM

If the patient becomes hyperthyroid while pregnant the hyperthyroidism must be brought under control as quickly as possible because otherwise there is a greater risk of spontaneous abortion. The most commonly used drug in Britain is carbimazole which if given in doses of 15 mg 8 hourly will usually result in the euthyroid state being reached in 4–6 weeks. From then on the dose can be progressively reduced, assessing the patient's clinical state and the FT_4I, until a maintenance dose of between 5 and 15 mg is reached. Hyperthyroidism can often be controlled with a lower dose of carbimazole during the last trimester than in the earlier stages of pregnancy. This might be due to the increased concentrations of TBG binding the excess thyroid hormone produced.

An alternative method of treatment is to give a rather larger maintenance dose of carbimazole (5 mg q.i.d.) to ensure that the hyperthyroidism is kept absolutely under control and then to give the mother supplementary L-thyroxine to make sure that she does not become hypothyroid. The dose of L-thyroxine can be regulated by FT_4I measurements but is usually in the region of 0·3 mg each morning. Since the carbimazole administered to the mother readily crosses the placenta it will have an effect on the fetal thyroid, blocking thyroid hormone synthesis. However, hypothyroidism does not occur since enough of the thyroxine administered to the mother crosses the placenta to keep the fetus euthyroid. On my unit we routinely sample cord blood in order to make sure the neonate's thyroid hormone levels are normal.

After delivery the mother should not breast feed her baby since carbimazole is secreted in breast milk.

SURGICAL TREATMENT

Partial thyroidectomy has been recommended as the treatment of choice for hyperthyroidism in pregnancy, particularly during the middle trimester when the risk of obstetric complications is relatively low (Becker and Sudduth, 1959; Hawe and Francis, 1962). However, generally speaking women of child bearing age are the ones most likely to go into remission on drug therapy, between 50 and 60% of them remaining euthyroid when drugs are stopped after $1\frac{1}{2}$ to 2 years' treatment (Montgomery and Welbourn, 1975). Partial thyroidectomy should be recommended however for those who co-operate badly while on medical therapy, those with large goitres and pressure symptoms, those who have allergies to all the usual antithyroid drugs and those who for geographical reasons find it hard to attend for careful control of the thyroid state during pregnancy. 35% of patients after partial thyroidectomy become hypothyroid for a few months until the thyroid remnant has hypertrophied (Toft et al., 1976) and for this reason it is advisable to follow the patient post-operatively with estimations of the FT_4I or to place her arbitrarily on adequate L-thyroxine to maintain a normal FT_4I, which is usually 0·2–0·3 mg per day. A baby born of a mother who has been allowed to go hypothyroid during pregnancy is much more likely itself to be born hypothyroid. Possibly what happens is that the mother's high TBG encourages the placental transfer of thyroid hormones from fetus to mother.

OUTCOME OF PREGNANCY

In my personal series all the 17 babies born of 16 mothers with hyper-thyroidism treated medically were born alive. The mean gestation was 40 weeks, the same as that of a control group of 46 women with no evidence of thyroid disease. Similarly the median Apgar score of 9 was the same as that of controls. The mean birthweight of 2930 g was significantly lower than those of controls (3490 g).

There was no significant increase in obstetric complications in the babies of mothers being treated for hyperthyroidism compared with the controls. One baby when mother received propyl thiouracil instead of carbimazole, because of a drug reaction to the latter, was born with a small goitre. The cord TSH was elevated, but both the FT_4I and the FT_3I were close to the median values of the control babies. The baby was euthyroid clinically, the goitre disappeared within a few weeks and the child has developed quite normally. It is believed that, in addition to an effect on hormone synthesis in the thyroid gland, propyl thiouracil has some inhibitory action on the peripheral deiodination of T_4 to T_3. Since T_3 is the more metabolically active of the two hormones this may have led to a less efficient feedback control of TSH and allowed a goitre to develop.

One other baby had a persistent vitelline duct and another had an inguinal hernia. It is not possible to say whether these abnormalities were related to carbimazole therapy. Both mothers were receiving the drug at the time of conception.

NEONATAL HYPERTHYROIDISM

Neonatal hyperthyroidism is usually regarded as a rare condition. However, in my series of 27 mothers with either hyperthyroidism during pregnancy or a previous history of Graves' disease two mothers gave birth to babies who developed thyrotoxicosis in the neonatal period, a prevalence of 7·4%. Moreover, one of the mothers had lost two previous babies because of intrauterine and neonatal thyrotoxicosis (Ramsay, 1976). She had thyrotoxicosis treated at the age of 11 by thyroidectomy. By the age of 16 she was hypothyroid and was placed on L-thyroxine. At the age of 21 she lost a baby at 28 weeks' gestation. It had a goitre and cardiac hypertrophy. Her second baby was born at 36 weeks' gestation. By the second day of life it became apparent that it was suffering from neonatal thyrotoxicosis and treatment was initiated. However, the baby died on the 4th day. At postmortem there was a goitre and cardiac hypertrophy. When she became pregnant for the third time she was recognized as being at considerable risk for having a third baby with thyrotoxicosis. She was therefore, in addition to 0·3 mg of thyroxine, given carbimazole during pregnancy, in order to control the fetal thyroid. This was successful; the baby was born at a normal weight and the cord blood thyroid hormone concentrations were normal. However, the next day at a time when the effect of maternal carbimazole had worn off the baby developed the signs of thyrotoxicosis and was promptly treated, with a good outcome. The mother's blood contained a high concentration of the thyroid stimulating immunoglobulin called long-acting thyroid stimulator-protector (LATS-P) which has been shown to be invariably present in the blood of mothers who give birth to babies with neonatal thyrotoxicosis (Dirmikis and Munro, 1975). It passes across the placenta and remains in the blood of the baby for several weeks after birth. Thus neonatal thyrotoxicosis is a self limiting disease and so long as the hyperthyroidism is adequately controlled in the first 2 or 3 weeks after birth the outcome should be good. Without treatment the mortality is 12% (Samuel *et al.*, 1971). For this reason in my hospital all babies born of mothers with past or present Graves' disease are observed by the paediatricians for the first few days of life in order that the diagnosis may be made and treatment instituted early. Carbimazole alone may be sufficient in the mild to moderate case, but iodine should be used in addition in the severely affected baby.

It is to be hoped that by measuring thyroid stimulating immunoglobulins in the blood of pregnant women with Graves' disease, it may be possible to predict those whose babies are likely to develop neonatal thyrotoxicosis (Dirmikis and Munro, 1975).

HYPOTHYROIDISM

Hypothyroidism tends to cause menorrhagia and infertility but women with mild hypothyroidism can become pregnant and in them there is a higher rate of spontaneous abortion, stillbirth and mental and physical abnormality in the babies than in the normal population (Greenman *et al.*, 1962; Jones and Man, 1969; Man *et al.*, 1971). For this reason it is important to look for hypothyroidism in women with menorrhagia or infertility and to detect it early in those who are pregnant. The most useful clinical features in the pregnant woman are cold intolerance and diminished sweating, a slow pulse rate and delayed relaxation of the ankle jerks. Measurement of the FT_4I will show that it is diminished. If the FT_4I is close to the lower limit of normal it is worth while estimating TSH since in primary hypothyroidism this will be elevated owing to the lack of feedback control by thyroid hormones on the hypothalamus and pituitary.

Treatment consists of replacement therapy with L-thyroxine. As there is little danger of ischaemic heart disease in women during the reproductive years, the dose can be built up fairly rapidly, though it is best to be more cautious if there is evidence of congenital or rheumatic heart disease. Normally one can start with 0·1 mg per day, increasing to 0·2 mg per day after a week. The dosage is adjusted until the FT_4I is in the middle of the normal range. A more sophisticated technique is to increase the dose of L-thyroxine until the serum TSH is suppressed into the normal range.

If a mother has previously given birth to an athyrotic cretin it is probably wise to give the mother enough thyroxine, as soon as pregnancy is diagnosed, to push the FT_4I up to a level which is at the upper limit of normal, since, as has already been shown, the thyroxine should cross the placenta and be able to maintain normal thyroid hormone concentrations in the fetus. There are some (Fisher, 1975) who disagree with this view and believe that it is necessary to inject the fetus intramuscularly with thyroid hormones or to inject them into the amniotic fluid. However, little information is available about the effectiveness of either of these approaches (van Herle *et al.*, 1975).

COLLOID GOITRE

A goitre is present in up to 70% of pregnant women in Britain (Crooks *et al.*, 1964). In most of them it will be very small and will require no treatment. The goitre is due to relative iodine deficiency, since in a country such as Iceland which has a high iodine intake there is no increase in the prevalence of goitre during pregnancy (Crooks *et al.*, 1967). It might seem reasonable therefore, in a woman with a family history of colloid goitre or in a patient who has had a goitre in previous pregnancies, to give supplementary iodine. This is most easily done by using iodized salt (1 part per 40 000) in cooking and on food. If this is unsuccessful, or the goitre is already large, thyroxine therapy during pregnancy will either reduce the size of the goitre or at least prevent it from becoming larger. The usual dose is 0·2–0·3 mg and excessive dosage can be prevented by monitoring the FT_4I.

NODULAR GOITRE

Nodular goitres discovered for the first time in pregnancy pose more of a problem. If the goitre contains several nodules and there is a family history of goitre it is most likely that the patient has a multinodular goitre, particularly if the nodules are firm but not hard and are relatively smooth. Thyroid isotope scanning should of course not be carried out during pregnancy, though, if it has been carried out inadvertently during pregnancy and technecium has been used, there is no fear for the fetus since technecium involves a radiation dose which is 150 times less than that of ^{131}I and is half the radiation dose given by a chest X-ray.

If there is a solitary nodule in the thyroid it is important to make sure that it is not an autonomous hyperfunctioning adenoma. This can be diagnosed by estimating FT_4I and FT_3I in the blood. The latter is especially important since the adenoma may only be producing excess T_3 and not T_4, a state known as 'T_3 toxicosis' (Marsden *et al.*, 1975).

We have found thyroid ultrasound to be useful in the diagnosis of a solitary nodule in the thyroid and of course, this is a harmless procedure in pregnancy (Ramsay and Meire, 1975). It tells us whether the nodule is solid or cystic. If it is cystic it may be worth aspirating the cyst and sending the aspirate for cytology (Crile and Hawk, 1973). Usually they turn out to be benign. The nodule which shows a solid pattern on ultrasound is more of a problem, since there is a greater chance of it being malignant. If the nodule is hard or fixed to other structures in the neck, if there are palpable lymph nodes or symptoms such as hoarseness or dysphagia, the thyroid should be operated on without delay. If none of these features is present it is justifiable to keep the nodule under review and only do something if it appears to be enlarging. Drill biopsy of the thyroid can be performed safely under local anaesthetic and may provide the diagnosis.

HASHIMOTO'S THYROIDITIS

Hashimoto's thyroiditis may rarely present in pregnancy. The patient may give a history of the recent onset of a goitre which may be tender. On palpation the goitre is hard and irregular, but not fixed. The patient may be clinically euthyroid or hypothyroid, so that the FT_4I may not necessarily be of any help. In almost all cases the thyroid antibodies will be strongly positive and will provide the diagnosis. Treatment with L-thyroxine is indicated since even the euthyroid ones will eventually become hypothyroid. Thyroxine therapy frequently will reduce the size of the goitre.

ACKNOWLEDGEMENTS

I would like to thank Dr S. Kaur and Dr G. Krassas for their help, Dr Stuart McHardy-Young for T_3 and TSH assays and Mrs Janet Howe for the statistical calculations.

References

Astwood, E. B. (1951). The use of antithyroid drugs during pregnancy. *J. Clin. Endocrinol.*, **11**, 1045

Becker, W. F. and Sudduth, P. G. (1959). Hyperthyroidism and pregnancy. *Ann. Surg.*, **149**, 867

Chopra, I. J., Sack, J. and Fisher, D. A. (1975). Reverse T_3 in the fetus and newborn. In D. A. Fisher and G. N. Burrow (eds.) *Perinatal Thyroid Physiology and Disease*, pp. 33–48. (New York: Raven Press)

Crile, G., Jr. and Hawk, W. A. (1973). Aspiration biopsy of thyroid nodules. *Surg. Gynecol. Obstet.*, **136**, 241

Crooks, J., Aboul-Khair, S. A., Turnbull, A. C. and Hytten, F. E. (1964). The incidence of goitre during pregnancy. *Lancet*, **ii**, 334

Crooks, J., Tulloch, M. I., Turnbull, A. C., Davidsson, D., Skulason, T. and Snaedal, G. (1967). Comparative incidence of goitre in pregnancy in Iceland and Scotland. *Lancet*, **ii**, 625

Dirmikis, S. M. and Munro, D. S. (1975). Placental transmission of thyroid stimulating immunoglobulins. *Br. Med. J.*, **2**, 665

Dussault, J., Row, V. V., Lickrish, G. and Volpé, R. (1969). Studies of serum triiodothyronine concentration in maternal and cord blood: transfer of triiodothyronine across the human placenta. *J. Clin. Endocrinol. Metab.*, **29**, 595

Erenburg, A., Phelps, D. L., Lam, R. and Fisher, D. A. (1974). Total and free thyroid hormone concentrations in the neonatal period. *Pediatrics*, **53**, 211

Fisher, D. A. (1975). Reverse triiodothyronine and fetal thyroid status. *N. Engl. J. Med.*, **293**, 770

Fisher, D. A. and Odell, W. D. (1969). Acute release of thyrotropin (TSH) in the newborn. *Pediatr. Res.*, **3**, 378

Goolden, A. W. G., Gartside, J. M. and Sanderson, C. (1967). Thyroid status in pregnancy and in women taking oral contraceptives. *Lancet*, **i**, 12

Greenberg, A. H., Czernichow, P., Reba, R. C., Tyson, J. and Blizzard, R. M. (1970). Observations on the maturation of thyroid function in early fetal life. *J. Clin. Invest.*, **49**, 1790

Greenman, G. W., Gabrielson, M. O., Howard-Flanders, J. and Wessel, M. A. (1962). Thyroid dysfunction in pregnancy. Fetal loss and follow-up evaluation of surviving infants. *N. Engl. J. Med.*, **267**, 426

Grumbach, M. M. and Werner, S. L. (1956). Transfer of thyroid hormone across the human placenta at term. *J. Clin. Endocrinol. Metab.*, **16**, 1392

Hawe, P. and Francis, H. H. (1962). Pregnancy and thyrotoxicosis. *Br. Med. J.*, **ii**, 817

van Herle, A. J., Young, R. T., Fisher, D. A., Allen, R. P. and Brinkman, C. R. (1975). Intra-uterine treatment of a hypothyroid fetus. *J. Clin. Endocrinol. Metab.*, **40**, 474

Javert, C. T. (1940). Hyperthyroidism and pregnancy. *Am. J. Obstet. Gynecol.*, **39**, 954

Jones, W. S. and Man, E. B. (1969). Thyroid function in human pregnancy. VI. Premature deliveries and reproductive failures of pregnant women with low serum butanol-extractable iodines. Maternal serum TBG and TBPA capacities. *Am. J. Obstet. Gynecol.*, **104**, 909

Kibel, I. (1944). Hyperthyroidism and pregnancy. *Am. J. Obstet. Gynecol.*, **48**, 553

Lieblich, J. M. and Utiger, R. D. (1973). Triiodothyronine in cord serum. *J. Pediatr.*, **82**, 290

Logan, W. P. D. and Cushion, A. A. (1958). Studies on medical and population subjects (No. 14). *Morbidity Statistics from General Practice, Vol. I. General.* (London: Her Majesty's Stationery Office)

Man, E. B., Holden, R. H. and Jones, W. S. (1971). Thyroid function in human pregnancy. VII. Development and retardation of 4-year-old progeny of euthyroid and of hypothyroxinemic women. *Am. J. Obstet. Gynecol.*, **109**, 12

Marsden, P., Facer, P., Acosta, M. and McKerron, C. G. (1975). Serum triiodothyronine in solitary autonomous nodules of the thyroid. *Clin. Endocrinol.*, **4**, 327

Montalvo, J. M., Wahner, H. W., Mayberry, W. E. and Lum, R. K. (1973). Serum tri-iodothyronine, total thyroxine, and thyroxine to triiodothyronine ratios in paired maternal-cord sera and at one week and one month of age. *Pediatr. Res.*, **7**, 706

Montgomery, D. A. D. and Welbourn, R. B. (1975). *Medical and Surgical Endocrinology*, p. 299. (London: Edward Arnold)

Ramsay, I. (1976). Attempted prevention of neonatal thyrotoxicosis. *Br. Med. J.* (In press)

Ramsay, I. and Meire, H. (1975). Ultrasonics in the diagnosis of thyroid disease. *Clin. Radiol.*, **26**, 191

Ramsay, I., Kaur, S. and Krassas, G. (1976). Hyperthyroidism in pregnancy; the outcome of combined antithyroid and thyroxine therapy. (In preparation)

Samuel, S., Pildes, R. S., Lewison, M. and Rosenthal, I. M. (1971). Neonatal hyperthyroidism in an infant born of a euthyroid mother. *Am. J. Dis. Child.*, **121**, 440

Toft, A. D., Irvine, W. J., McIntosh, D., Seth, J., Cameron, E. H. D. and Lidgard, G. P. (1976). Temporary hypothyroidism after surgical treatment of thyrotoxicosis. *Lancet*, **ii**, 817

Tunbridge, W. M. G. and Hall, R. (1975). Thyroid function in pregnancy. In F. E. Hytten (ed.) *Physiological Adjustments in Pregnancy. Clinics in Obstetrics and Gynaecology*, Vol. 2, No. 2. (New York and London: W. B. Saunders)

Tunbridge, W. M. G., Evered, D. C., Hall, R., Appleton, D., Brewis, M., Clark, F., Grimley Evans, J., Young, E., Bird, T. and Smith, P. (1976). The prevalence of thyroid disorders in an English community. In J. Robbins and L. E. Braverman (eds.) *Thyroid Research; Proceedings of the Seventh International Thyroid Conference.* Boston, Mass, June 9–13, 1975. (Amsterdam: Excerpta Medica)

Discussion

Lloyd, G., London: What is the evidence that there is an increased thyroid binding globulin during pregnancy? Are you measuring TBG directly?

Ramsay: I have not measured thyroid binding globulin directly. My evidence for it being increased comes from the results of the T_3 resin uptake test. However, others have measured it directly and the level of TBG doubles during pregnancy.

Essex, Nina: If you treat a patient surgically for thyrotoxicosis and then give them oral thyroxine do you increase the chances of the patient becoming hypothyroid subsequently?

Ramsay: No, I do not think so. All you are doing is delaying the TSH mediated hypertrophy of the thyroid. I do not think this matters. So far as the pregnant patient is concerned I think it better to wait until the pregnancy is over. It is my impression that if a woman is hypothyroid during pregnancy then she may come to depend on the thyroxine from the normal infant. The increased maternal TBG can attract thyroxine from the fetus across the placenta and lower the level in the baby. There is no direct evidence of this but it seems a theoretical possibility. This might account for the increase in congenital defects in babies from mothers with hypothyroidism.

9
The Drug Treatment of Epilepsy in Pregnancy

A. HOPKINS

'The drug treatment of epilepsy in pregnancy'—is a specific and clear title but unfortunately rather limiting in scope, particularly since Dr Roy Meadow discusses an important area in the next chapter. I propose, therefore, to expand my subject into the following areas.

1. Should a woman with epilepsy have children?

2. Is epilepsy particularly prone to start during pregnancy?

3. If already present, do seizures become more or less frequent during pregnancy?

4. What variations are there in the pharmacology of anticonvulsant drugs during pregnancy?

5. What risk is there of the administration of anticonvulsants to the mother resulting in intoxication of the child, either via the placenta, or via the milk?

6. How should status epilepticus be treated during pregnancy, and why is there a difference in the drugs used for treating status and eclampsia?

Should a woman with epilepsy have children?

Until about 30 years ago it was believed that a major factor in the causation of epilepsy was the genetic endowment. Belief in the 'epileptic constitution' led, in the case of some states of America and in Scandinavian countries, to the promulgation of laws banning the marriage of those with epilepsy. There undoubtedly is a genetic component, but the following argument, derived from Metrakos and Metrakos (1974) shows the difficulty of proving it. Assume that epilepsy is *entirely* due to the interaction of only three genes, one dominant A, and two recessive b, c. An epileptic proband may therefore be Aa, bb, cc or AA, bb, cc. For the first example parents could be Aa, Bb, Cc and aa, Bb, Cc. Although the first parent (say the mother) carries A, this is not expressed, as she—and in fact her husband as well—are heterozygous for b and c. The risk that a sibling of the proband will also have the genotype Aa, bb, cc is only 1/32. If we assume that penetrance is as high as 80%, then this chance falls to $1/32 \times 0.8$. But the variation of expression with age must also be considered. This is further discussed below, but for the moment it would be reasonable to assume at any age an expression of 30%. The chances of a second sibling being affected therefore falls to $1/32 \times 0.8 \times 0.3 = 0.0075$, or one chance in 133. As the prevalence of epilepsy is one in 200, it can be seen that quite modest assumptions can fully account for the occurrence of epilepsy on an entirely genetic basis, and yet we know that, taking a sample of people with epilepsy in the community, the risk of an epileptic adult having a child with epilepsy is only about one chance in 40. This disparity has been largely explained by the work of Metrakos and Metrakos in Montreal over the last 15 years. They have shown that the siblings and parents of those with centrencephalic epilepsy—that is to say epilepsy with 3 Hz spike and wave discharges—also have a very high probability of having similar electroencephalographic discharges (and a lesser probability of overt seizures) although this probability varies greatly with age. The siblings and parents of those probands with epilepsy of other types do not have, broadly speaking, an increased probability of having either abnormal electro-encephalograms or seizures. It follows that correct genetic counselling depends on an accurate clinical and electroencephalographic classification of the seizure type(s) of the potential parents.

Is epilepsy particularly prone to start during pregnancy?

The age-specific annual incidence rate for epilepsy is roughly constant at about 40/100 000 throughout the childbearing period. Pregnancy and the onset of non-eclamptic seizures will therefore coincide by chance alone in a number of women. Although there are some women whose first (of many) seizures occurred in pregnancy, I know of no study which provides statistical evidence that supports a view that pregnancy is likely to 'start' epilepsy. A rather different problem is non-eclamptic seizures which occur for the first time in pregnancy, remit in the puerperium, and then return only in subsequent pregnancies. Knight and Rhind (1975) have collected only two such patients out of their 59 epileptic mothers studied through 153 pregnancies. Furthermore it is rare, in a case of pre-existing epilepsy, for seizures to recur during pregnancy after a prolonged seizure-free period. The apparent rarity of these phenomena suggests that pregnancy *per se* is not a particularly potent epileptogenic agent. Finally, an isolated single non-eclamptic seizure may occur during pregnancy; it is reasonable to withhold anticonvulsants in such cases, beginning such drugs only if subsequent seizures occur.

104

If the onset of epilepsy has preceded pregnancy, do seizures tend to become more or less frequent during pregnancy?

Knight and Rhind (1975) list nine studies on this topic dating from 1889 which show an enormous variatio.ı in results. In their study, 45% of their women had an increased frequency in seizures during pregnancy and 5% a decreased frequency, whilst in the immediately preceding study (1970) only 24% showed an increased frequency and 48% a decrease! These converse results may presumably in part be accounted for by a difference in patient selection, and different practices in anticonvulsant treatment. If we take the study of Knight and Rhind as being representative of recent British experience, the lessons that may be drawn are as follows:

1. 45% have more frequent seizures, 50% show no change, and 5% have a decreased frequency of seizures.

2. Whether the epilepsy is idiopathic or symptomatic does not make much difference to these figures. (This study however contains an excessively large number of mothers with so-called idiopathic epilepsy, suggesting that classification of seizures was not accurate.)

3. Those who have very frequent seizures (monthly or more frequently) are four times more likely to have an increased frequency of seizures during pregnancy than those with occasional seizures (less than one in three months).

4. Those who carry a male fetus are twice as likely to deteriorate than those carrying a female fetus. This rather surprising tendency has been found in two other studies (for references, see Knight and Rhind, 1975).

What are the reasons for the increase in frequency of seizures in some pregnant women with epilepsy?

1. The first point to note is that unexplained alterations in the frequency of seizures are commonplace in both men and non-pregnant women, so that an increase in frequency during pregnancy may be purely coincidental.

2. The general practitioner or obstetrician may reduce or stop anticonvulsants in an attempt to reduce the chances of the woman bearing an abnormal child (see Meadow's paper in this volume).

3. Compliance in taking medication may be less as the patient takes her own decision to reduce the chances of teratogenicity.

4. The weight gain of pregnancy will tend to dilute the oral dose of anticonvulsants if this is maintained at the level preceding conception.

5. It is known that water retention, artificially induced by pitressin may precipitate seizures in some susceptible individuals. It is possible that the water retention of pregnancy may have the same result.

6. It is well known amongst those interested in epilepsy that stress and other emotional factors may precipitate seizures. *A priori* one might expect such factors to be more dominant in pregnancy.

7. There may be some changes in the pharmacology of anticonvulsants in pregnancy (see next section).

What variations are there in the pharmacology of anticonvulsant drugs during pregnancy?

The serum levels of anticonvulsants can be measured by gas liquid chromatography, or by radioimmunoassay. The methods and pharmacokinetics of each drug has been reviewed by Richens (1976). The usual method for determining the rate of metabolism of a drug in an individual patient is to administer a single dose and follow the serum concentration serially subsequently. The half-life and clearance of the drug can then be calculated. Most drugs are cleared at a rate proportional to the concentration—so-called first-order kinetics. However, the hydroxylating enzyme which is responsible for metabolizing one of the most commonly used anticonvulsant drugs, phenytoin, to its principal metabolite 5(parahydroxyphenyl)-5-phenylhydantoin becomes saturated even at serum levels in the therapeutic range. If the enzyme has already reached its maximum rate of action, a small increment in dosage will have a large effect on the serum level. As might be expected, this system, operating in so-called zero order kinetics, is extremely sensitive to any factor which inhibits, blocks or competes with the hydroxylating enzyme, when the serum phenytoin will rise. Pheneturide, for example, causes an immediate rise in serum phenytoin if added to the anticonvulsant regime. Sulthiame causes a rise after an interval of some 20 days, perhaps by inhibiting the production of microsomal hydroxylating enzymes. Alternatively any factor which results in enzyme induction will cause more rapid hydroxylation of phenytoin. Phenytoin itself induces production of hydroxylating enzymes which are responsible for hydroxylating also sex hormones and vitamin D. Both failure of oral contraception (Janz and Schmidt, 1974) and osteomalacia (Richens and Rowe, 1970) have been reported on this account.

What, then, happens in pregnancy? There is only one small study published (Sherwin et al., 1974). These workers report that plasma phenytoin levels did not change much in pregnancy, though some pregnant women had slightly, but insignificantly, lower levels supporting this finding. A criticism of this study is that all the reported levels were below the lower limit of the generally accepted range. A further unpublished study (Landon and Kirkley, 1976) and another unpublished study by Dam and co-workers (communication to A. Richens, 1976), suggests that pregnancy is associated with increased induction of hydroxylating enzymes with a consequent fall in the serum levels of the two drugs studied (carbamazepine and phenytoin). Shortly after delivery Dam and co-workers found that there is a sharp reversal in this process so that, if these drugs had been increased during pregnancy, toxic serum levels would result. The administration of phenytoin also results in a reduction of serum, red cell and cerebrospinal fluid folate in the great majority of cases. The suggested mechanisms of this are reviewed by Richens (1976). It is probable that induction of folate metabolizing enzymes is responsible. Although it has been claimed that the administration of folic acid, to correct this deficiency, may result in aggravation of the epilepsy, the majority view is that the evidence for this is slight. If a pregnant women taking phenytoin has a folate deficient megaloblastic anaemia, it would seem reasonable for her to have supplements of folic acid — and vitamin D as well.

What is the risk of the administration of anticonvulsants crossing the placenta, or into breast milk?

The placental transmission of anticonvulsants is reviewed in the following chapter by Meadows. There is virtually no work on entry to milk, but single observations by Coradello (1973) show no entry to the milk of mothers taking phenobarbitone, methyl phenobarbitone or phenytoin.

The treatment of status epilepticus in pregnancy, and comparison with the treatment of eclampsia

Influenced, perhaps, by the management of eclampsia, obstetricians tended to terminate pregnancy at once if status epilepticus supervened. Modern policy is to treat the patient as if not pregnant, and to attempt to control seizures with efficient use of parenteral medication, maintaining adequate arterial oxygenation if necessary by anaesthesia and intermittent positive pressure ventilation (IPPR). Status epilepticus of major seizures is a life threatening situation, and treatment should be undertaken in an intensive therapy unit. Present policy is to use an intravenous benzodiazepine (diazepam or clonazepam) as a drug of first choice. Experience is greater with diazepam. The first step is an intravenous injection of 10 mg in 2 ml over 3 minutes, followed if necessary, which is rare, by a further 5–10 mg in 5 minutes. Significant respiratory depression and hypotension will follow in some cases. The anticonvulsant effect may be short lived, in which case a solution containing 100–200 mg should be set up and infused at a rate of approximately 100 ml/h, reducing as the seizures come under control. If this fails, then the patient should be treated with intravenous thiopentone (Brown and Horton, 1967). Respiratory depression is almost certain with this drug in adequate dosage and IPPR will be necessary. If the seizures are controlled early and adequate oxygenation has been maintained, there is no reason why the pregnancy should not go to term.

Diazepam has also been used successfully in the treatment of eclampsia (Lean *et al.*, 1968). Few units however can hope to rival the experience of Parklands, Dallas, Texas, where Pritchard and Pritchard (1975) have reported 154 cases of eclampsia without a single maternal death. Their cases were treated using, with hydrallazine, standard doses of magnesium sulphate, a drug unknown in clinical neurology, though perhaps neurologists should be using it. Magnesium inhibits release of acetyl choline from presynaptic terminals, and potentiates blockade produced by decamethonium, d-tubocurarine and succinylcholine. It has been shown that, if slowly infused, serum levels may be reached which result in complete paralysis in the absence of anaesthesia (Somjen *et al.*, 1966).

Conclusion

The woman with epilepsy may be encouraged to have children as the risk of transmission is not great unless she, or her husband have 3 Hz spike and wave discharges on the electroencephalogram. Epilepsy is not particularly likely to start during pregnancy. It may be exacerbated by pregnancy, particularly if seizures were frequent before conception. This increase in frequency may well be due to induction, by pregnancy, of hydroxylating enzymes which lower the levels of anticonvulsant drugs. Those who deteriorate are more likely to be carrying a male fetus. Folic acid and vitamin D should be given throughout pregnancy. Status epilepticus should be treated vigorously by intravenous diazepam, maintaining adequate oxygenation. Anticonvulsants cross the placenta, but do not enter breast milk.

References

Brown, A. S. and Horton, J. M. (1967). Status epilepticus treated by intravenous infusion of thiopentone sodium. *Br. Med. J.*, **1**, 27

Coradello, H. (1973). Uber die Ausscheidung von Antiepileptika in die Muttermilch. *Wien. Klin. Wochensch.*, **85**, 695

Janz, D. and Schmidt, D. (1974). Antiepileptic drugs and failure of oral contraceptives. *Lancet*, i, 1113

Knight, A. H. and Rhind, E. G. (1975). Epilepsy and pregnancy: a study of 153 pregnancies in 59 patients. *Epilepsia*, **16**, 99

Lean, T. H., Ratnam, S. S. and Sivasambro, R. (1968). Use of benzodiazepines in the management of eclampsia. *J. Obstet. Gynaecol. Br. Commonw.*, **75**, 856

Metrakos, K. and Metrakos, J. D. (1974). Genetics of epilepsy. In P. J. Vinken and G. W. Bruyn (eds.) *Handbook of Clinical Neurology*. (Amsterdam: Elsevier)

Pritchard, J. A. and Pritchard, S. A. (1975). Standardized treatment of 154 consecutive cases of eclampsia. *Am. J. Obstet. Gynecol.*, **123**, 543

Richens, A. (1976). *Drug Treatment of Epilepsy*, p. 176. (London: Henry Kimpton)

Richens, A. and Rowe, D. J. F. (1970). Disturbance of calcium metabolism by anticonvulsant drugs. *Br. Med. J.*, **4**, 73

Sherwin, A. L., Loynd, J. S., Bock, G. W. and Sokolowski, C. D. (1974). Effects of age, sex, obesity, and pregnancy of plasma diphenylhydantoin levels. *Epilepsia*, **15**, 507

Somjen, G., Hilmy, M. and Stephen, C. R. (1966). Failure to anesthetize human subjects by intravenous administration of magnesium sulfate. *J. Pharmacol. Exp. Therapeut.*, **154**, 652

10
Epilepsy, Anticonvulsants and Abnormal Babies

S. R. MEADOW

In 1968 six infants with cleft lip and palate were reported who had been born to mothers who had taken anticonvulsants during pregnancy (Meadow, 1968). A request was made to doctors in Britain to notify abnormal babies who were born to mothers suffering from epilepsy. This resulted in the reporting of 32 children, 20 of whom had cleft lip and/or palate and eight of whom had congenital heart lesions (Meadow, 1970); 11 were noted to have a particular characteristic facial appearance. Analysis of the birth dates of the children, and the incidence of epilepsy in Britain suggested that more abnormal children had been born to epileptic mothers than would have been expected by chance. Moreover, all the mothers were taking anticonvulsant drugs during pregnancy. This suggested that anticonvulsants might be teratogenic, and raised the possibility that the antifolate activity of anti-convulsants was the mechanism.

Since then a large number of surveys have been completed. Though some facts have become clearly established, there are still many uncertainties.

THE OUTCOME OF PREGNANCY IN WOMEN WITH EPILEPSY

Table 10.1 shows the results of surveys of the incidence of congenital abnormalities in women with epilepsy. Some of the surveys have compared the incidence with that in matched control non-epileptic women, others have compared the incidence with the expected incidence of congenital abnor-malities in their region.

The difference in the malformation rate between the different surveys is largely accounted for by differences in the definition of a major mal-formation. However, it is clear that the incidence of malformation in babies

109

Table 10.1 The incidence of congenital anomalies in the children of women with epilepsy

Author(s)	Control group or population				Epileptic group			
	Number of births*	Malformation (%)	Cleft lip ±palate (%)	Heart anomalies (%)	Number of births*	Malformation (%)	Cleft lip ±palate (%)	Heart anomalies (%)
Speidel and Meadow, 1972	448	1·6	0·2	0·2	388	4·4	0·8	1·5
Watson and Spellacy, 1971	50	0	0	0	51	5·9	0	2·0
Elshove and van Eck, 1971	12051	1·9	0·26	N.S.	65	15·0	5·0	3·1
Fedrick, 1973	649	5·6	0	0·7	217	13·8	0·5	0·9
Koppe et al., 1973	12300	3·5	N.S.	N.S.	192	6·8	0·5	2·0
Lowe, 1973	31877	2·8	0·16	N.S.†	245	5·0	0·7	1·2
Millar and Nevin, 1973	32227	3·8	0·22	N.S.	110	6·4	1·8	N.S.
Niswander and Wertelecki, 1973	347097	2·7	0·15	N.S.	413	4·1	0·73	N.S.
Monson et al., 1973	50591	2·4	N.S.	N.S.	306	4·7	1·0	1·0
South, 1972	7896	2·4	0·2	N.S.	31	6·4	6·4	0
Bjerkeda and Bahna, 1973	125423	2·2	0·16	N.S.	371	4·5	1·8	N.S.

* Includes stillbirths as well as live births

† N.S. Not stated

born to epileptic mothers is increased by a factor of 2–3. Part of this increase is accounted for by the particularly high incidence of cleft lip and/or palate (10 times more likely) and congenital heart lesions (4 times more likely).

Apart from major malformations other abnormalities have been noted. Minor skeletal abnormalities were recorded in several of the early cases (Meadow, 1970). In 1970 it was found that hypoplasia of the terminal phalanges of the fingers was frequent, the ulna fingers being more affected than the radial (Loughran et al., 1973). This has been confirmed by others (Barry and Danks, 1974; Barr et al., 1974).

Many of the children born to epileptic mothers have a characteristic facial appearance, with wide-spaced eyes, low posterior hair line, short neck, prominent brow and trigoncephaly. Different authors have attempted to link a particular appearance with an individual drug (Hanson and Smith, 1975; Zackai et al., 1975). But others have observed a similar facial appearance from several different anticonvulsant drugs and it is doubtful if the appearance and abnormalities from one anticonvulsant are significantly different from another.

More worrying has been the report that the offspring are more likely to have retarded growth, delayed development and mental subnormality (Seip, 1976; Speidel and Meadow, 1972; Hill et al., 1974).

THE CAUSE OF THE ABNORMALITIES

There are many reasons why an epileptic mother might be considered to have an increased chance of an abnormal baby.

Teratogenic action of anticonvulsant drugs

Some of the surveys have contrasted the incidence of abnormalities in epileptic mothers not taking drugs with those taking anticonvulsant drugs. Table 10.2 shows that the increased malformation rate is confined to those mothers who took anticonvulsants during pregnancy. (It is obvious that the

Table 10.2 The malformation rate of babies exposed to anticonvulsants during pregnancy compared with those not exposed

Author(s)	Anticonvulsants		No anticonvulsants	
	Number of pregnancies	Malformation rate (%)	Number of pregnancies	Malformation rate (%)
Speidel and Meadow, 1972	329	5·2	59	0
Lowe, 1973	134	6·7	111	2·7
South, 1972	22	9·0	9	0
Janz and Fuchs, 1964	426	2·2	130	0
Koppe et al., 1973	125	8·8	67	3·0
Monson et al., 1973	205	5·3	101	2·9
Annegers et al., 1974	141	7·1	56	1·8

two groups are unlikely to contain women affected by similar severity of epilepsy; those who received drugs are more likely to have severe epilepsy.) From the table it emerges that the malformation rate in epileptic mothers not taking anticonvulsants is similar to the normal incidence, whereas it is raised in those who take anticonvulsants.

With regard to individual drugs, most authors suggest that phenytoin is the drug most commonly associated with congenital abnormalities, and that when combined with phenobarbitone the effect is even greater. But a great many drugs have been reported to have been associated with congenital malformations (Table 10.3) and the absence of certain more recently

Table 10.3   Anticonvulsant drugs reports to have been associated with congenital malformations

Phenytoin	Pheneturide
Phenobarbitone	Diazepam
Primidone	Troxidone (trimethadione)
Methylphenobarbitone	Paramethadione
Sulthiame	Ethosuximide
Phensuximide	Carbamazepine

developed drugs from that list may be related to the fact that they have not been used extensively for long enough. At this stage it would be unwise to state that 'drug x' is not associated with abnormalities. As with other drugs, teratogenetic activity occurs during the first trimester of pregnancy.

Anticonvulsant drugs readily cross the placenta (Mirkin, 1971; Melchior *et al.*, 1967) and, for example, the fetus is exposed to the same concentration of phenobarbitone as the mother. Little is known about the metabolism of phenytoin in human pregnancy but in rats its excretion is impaired and consequently maternal blood phenytoin levels are increased. In the mouse the malformation rate is directly related to the dosage and hence the blood levels. If a similar mechanism applied to the human, then a higher incidence of malformations would be expected in those patients taking large doses of anticonvulsants. However, no evidence was found that malformations were more common in a group of mothers taking large doses of phenytoin (Monson *et al.*, 1973). In another study a dosage effect for phenobarbitone was found, but not for phenytoin (Fedrick, 1973).

Although every agent found to be teratogenic in man has also been shown to be teratogenic in laboratory animals, findings in one species do not guarantee the same results in another and the risk in man can really only be determined in man.

Phenytoin has repeatedly been shown to cause cleft palate in Swiss Webster and A/Jax strains of mice (Massey, 1966; Harbison and Becker, 1969; Elshove, 1969, 1970). A variety of other malformations, particularly skeletal, also occur and the type of malformation depends upon the stage of pregnancy at which the phenytoin is given. The effect is also dose related, and indeed a single dose given at the right time (at 10 to 15 days) can produce a variety of fetal abnormalities. None of these malformations occurs spontaneously in the strains of mice studied, although the mouse is known to be peculiarly susceptible to teratogenic drugs.

The most popular hypothesis to account for the teratogenic action of anticonvulsants is their interference with folic acid metabolism. Folic acid plays an important role in the metabolism of the developing embryo. Folate antagonists such as aminopterin are known to cause malformations in the human and it is suspected, although the evidence is not conclusive, that folate deficiency is also teratogenic in man.

Anticonvulsants of the phenytoin and barbiturate groups are known to cause folic acid deficiency in epileptic patients (Malpas *et al.*, 1966). The present hypothesis is that the administration of certain anticonvulsants results in folate deficiency; when the further demands for folate which occur in early pregnancy are superimposed upon this deficiency a significant degree of impairment in folate supplies might occur at a critical stage of embryogenesis and result in malformation. Such a situation would be uncommon in the absence of a predisposing cause for low maternal folate levels. It has been suggested that folic acid has a protective effect on the teratogenic action of phenytoin as the frequency of cleft palate in mice was found to be lower with combined phenytoin-folic-acid administration than with phenytoin alone (Elshove, 1970). However, others have been unable to confirm such a protective effect.

There are many other ways in which anticonvulsants will affect the fetus. Phenytoin, for instance, has a wide variety of side-effects. It alters collagen breakdown and production, affects induction of many enzymes, stimulates the adrenal cortex and increases corticosteroid metabolism. There are reports of anticonvulsants causing disruption to chromosomes.

Genetic factors

It is possible that the genetic background that predisposes to idiopathic epilepsy also predisposes towards a woman (or man) producing a malformed child. Dronamraju (1970) reported that 17 to 20% of his patients with cleft lip with or without cleft palate had a first or second degree relative with epilepsy, and suggested that there may be a genetic relationship between epilepsy and cleft lip and palate. Moreover, the possibility exists that this relationship may extend to other malformations. Congenital heart disease is found in 5% of children with cleft lip with or without cleft palate and these are also the most common major anomalies in the children of epileptics.

Persons with severe epilepsy have a limited choice of spouse. Many marry other epileptics, so that the genetic contribution of paternal epilepsy may be important. Studies of the children of male epileptics have produced contradictory findings. A larger survey is needed.

Other factors

The severity of the epilepsy and frequency of fits during pregnancy does not seem to be related to the development of a malformed baby (Fedrick, 1972).

Although both severe epilepsy and congenital malformations do occur more commonly amongst the lower socio-economic groups, it can be shown that the increased incidence of malformation in the babies of epileptic mothers is independent of socio-economic factors (Monson *et al.*, 1973; Fedrick, 1972). In one survey a higher incidence of malformation was found in the pregnancies of the upper socio-economic group of epileptic mothers than the rest (Hill, 1973).

OTHER ADVERSE EFFECTS OF ANTICONVULSANTS ON THE FETUS

Many minor effects upon the fetus have been measured, but the most dangerous effect has been the occurrence of severe fetal haemorrhage. This is a rare occurrence but may be fatal (Mountain *et al.*, 1970). It is corrected by giving vitamin K to the mother during the last part of pregnancy. This is worthwhile because lethal fetal haemorrhage may occur during the last few weeks of pregnancy as well as during the first few days of life.

MANAGEMENT TO PREVENT FETAL ABNORMALITIES

Although it is highly probable that anticonvulsants are teratogenic and increase the chance of a major congenital abnormality by a factor of nearly 3, it would be unwise to stop giving anticonvulsants to epileptic women who need those drugs. At the present time, no one anticonvulsant drug has emerged as definitely safe for the fetus. But very large numbers of reports have emerged about the possible dangers of phenytoin.

Enough folic acid should be given during pregnancy (particularly during the first trimester) to maintain normal folic acid levels. The fact that malformation occurs during the first few weeks means that the epileptic mother would need to be receiving extra folate from the time of conception.

There is a case for advocating the inclusion of a small amount of folate in the anticonvulsant drugs given to women of childbearing age. Although large amounts of folate may affect control of epilepsy, it is most unlikely that small amounts would.

The woman with epilepsy has an increased chance of an abnormal baby and should be delivered in a hospital which has a neonatal service that can deal with the emergency.

Because of the occasional severe fetal or neonatal haemorrhage, vitamin K should be given to the mother in a dose of 10 mg a day orally during the last 2 months of pregnancy. At birth, 1 mg should be given by intramuscular injection to the baby.

114

During the neonatal period the baby should be examined with extra thoroughness because of the increased chance of congenital abnormality.

Women with epilepsy should be given genetic counselling so that they may judge the risks themselves. For some families in whom there is already a tendency to produce a particular abnormality, epilepsy and anticonvulsant drugs may increase the risk of that abnormality to an unacceptable degree.

References

Barr, M., Posnanski, A. K. and Schmickel, R. D. (1974). Digital hypoplasia and anticonvulsants during gestation: a teratogenic syndrome? *J. Paediatr.*, **84**, 254

Barry, J. E. and Danks, D. M. (1974). Anticonvulsants and congenital abnormalities. *Lancet*, **ii**, 48

Dronamraju, K. R. (1970). Epilepsy and cleft lip and palate. *Lancet*, **ii**, 876

Elshove, J. (1969). Cleft palate in the offspring of female mice treated with phenytoin. *Lancet*, **ii**, 1074

Elshove, J. (1970). Teratogene werking van fenytoine. Thesis, University of Gronigen

Fedrick, J. (1973). Epilepsy and pregnancy: a report from the Oxford Record Linkage Study. *Br. Med. J.*, **ii**, 442

Hanson, J. W. and Smith, D. W. (1975). The fetal hydantoin syndrome. *J. Paediatr.*, **87**, No. 2, 285

Harbison, R. D. and Becker, B. A. (1969). Relation of dosage and time of administration of diphenylhydantoin to its teratogenic effect in mice. *Teratology*, **2**, 305

Hill, R. M. (1973). Drugs ingested by pregnant women. *Clin. Pharmacol. Ther.*, **14**, 654

Hill, R. M., Verniaud, W. M., Horning, M. G., McCulley, L. B. and Morgan, N. F. (1974). Infants exposed in utero to antiepileptic drugs. *Am. J. Dis. Child.*, **127**, 645

Loughran, P. M., Gold, H. and Vance, J. C. (1973). Phenytoin teratogenicity in man. *Lancet*, **i**, 70

Malpas, J. S., Spray, G. A. and Witts, L. J. (1966). Serum folic acid and vitamin B_{12} levels in anticonvulsant therapy. *Br. Med. J.*, **1**, 955

Massey, K. M. (1966). Teratogenic effects of diphenylhydantoin sodium. *J. Oral Ther. Pharmacol.*, **2**, 380

Meadow, S. R. (1968). Anticonvulsant drugs and congenital abnormalities. *Lancet*, **ii**, 1296

Meadow, S. R. (1970). Congenital abnormalities and anticonvulsant drugs. *Proc. R. Coll. Med.*, **63**, 48

Melchior, J. C., Svensmark, O. and Trolle, D. (1967). Placental transfer of phenobarbitone in epileptic women and elimination in newborns. *Lancet*, **ii**, 860

Mirkin, B. L. (1971). Diphenylhydantoin. Placental transport, fetal localization, neonatal metabolism and possible teratogenic effects. *J. Paediatr.*, **78**, 329

Monson, R. R., Rosenburg, L., Hartz, S. C., Shapiro, S., Heinonen, O. P. and Slone, D. (1973). Diphenylhydantoin and selected congenital malformations. *N. Engl. J. Med.*, **289**, 1049

Mountain, K. R., Hirsh, J. and Gallus, A. S. (1970). Neonatal coagulation defect due to anticonvulsant drug treatment in pregnancy. *Lancet*, **i**, 265

Seip, M. (1976). Growth retardation, dysmorphic facies and minor malformations following exposure to phenobarbitone in utero. *Acta Paediatr. Scand.*, **65**, 617

Speidel, B. D. and Meadow, S. R. (1972). Maternal epilepsy and abnormalities of the foetus and newborn. *Lancet*, **ii**, 839

Zackai, E. H., Mellman, W. J., Neiderer, B. and Hanson, J. W. (1975). The fetal trimethadione syndrome. *J. Paediatr.*, **87**, No. 2, 280

Joint discussion

Dewhurst, C. J., London: Dr Hopkins, may I say that I am grateful to you for confirming a pearl of wisdom which I first heard many years ago at this hospital from the late Fred Gibberd. He taught me that when epileptics become pregnant some get better, some get worse and some stay the same. I am pleased to learn that this is still substantially true. Could I put to you a point which Dr Meadow made, that it would seem a sensible precaution to add folic acid to anticonvulsants, and phenytoin in particular, in the hope that this might prevent fetal malformation.

Hopkins: The problem with this suggestion is that there is some evidence that the administration of folate increases fit frequency in epileptics. This is a point of view put forward by Dr Reynolds of the Maudsley Hospital and is an opinion held by a body of research workers in the United States. This work has been criticized and I think I might say that it is still an open question. It is my own view that the congenital malformations attributed to anticonvulsants are probably related to abnormalities of connective tissue growth. Phenytoin and phenobarbitone to a lesser extent produce considerable abnormalities in connective tissue growth in children and young adults. I recall a striking instance recently of two sets of identical twins. One of each pair was on anticonvulsants. In each case the coarsening of the facial features in the treated twin was very apparent and this feature is well known to many of us who visit epileptic colonies. The administration of anticonvulsants during the growth years causes a general overgrowth of collagen in the gums, the lips and the cheek bones, producing a coarse facial appearance and I cannot help thinking that this abnormality is related in some way to the situation in the fetus.

Asfeldt, J. V., Canada: I was not clear what the expected incidence of epilepsy would be in the offspring of epileptic mothers?

Hopkins: The overall risk in a population of epileptic women is that their offspring will have one chance in 40 of having a non-febrile convulsion at some time in their lifetime. This is an increased level of risk and it is almost confined to the children of mothers with the idiopathic form of epilepsy.

11
Diabetic Therapy and Pregnancy

NINA ESSEX

With the advent of insulin the hazards of pregnancy to the diabetic mother were largely overcome. The perinatal mortality, however, remained alarmingly high for several years and despite a considerable fall over the last 25 years it is still twice as high as in a non-diabetic woman. Table 11.1 shows the perinatal mortality at King's College Hospital during the last 20 years.

Table 11.1 Perinatal mortality in diabetic pregnancies at KCH

| Years | Numbers of deliveries | Perinatal deaths | | Late deaths |
		Number	Percentage	
1951–55	132	42	32	
1956–60	180	30	17	
1961–65	213	24	11	3
1966–70	176	15	9	3
1971–75	173	6	4	1

During the years 1971–75 perinatal mortality was 3·5%. This compares with the national perinatal mortality of just below 2%.

The risks to the fetus are:

1. Increased stillbirth and neonatal death rate.

2. Excess intrauterine growth leading to possibility of obstructed vaginal delivery especially shoulder dystocia.

3. Increased perinatal morbidity especially hypoglycaemia and hyperbilirubinaemia.

4. Increased risk of congenital malformations.

The most obvious biochemical disturbance affecting the fetus of the diabetic woman is maternal hyperglycaemia. This is reflected by the fetus

117

whose blood glucose is approximately 1·5 mmol/l below the mother's except at very high levels of maternal blood glucose. The fetal pancreatic islets do not respond to the presence of glucose before the third trimester of pregnancy. After the 28th week they start to secrete insulin in response to a glucose stimulus and infants of diabetic mothers characteristically show an increased insulin response to a glucose load at birth compared with infants of normal mothers (Baird and Farquhar, 1962). This increased insulin response, presumably reflecting raised basal insulin secretion, is thought to be responsible for the excess fetal weight which is mainly due to fat although all organs and tissues except for brain are overweight. This excess fetal weight does not occur in fetuses lacking an intact hypothalamo–pituitary axis (de Gasparo and Hoet, 1971). Other factors may also be involved. It is difficult to explain excessively large babies born to women with very mild diabetes requiring dietary treatment only and at King's the heaviest babies have been born to women with mild, apparently well controlled diabetes.

Fetal hyperinsulinism will also lead to hypoglycaemia in the neonatal period once the maternal glucose load is removed particularly if feeding is delayed or infrequent.

Unexplained intrauterine death is less common but does occur occasionally. In the diabetic on insulin maternal hypoglycaemia may be an important factor in intrauterine death although this has never been convincingly demonstrated. If the mother becomes suddenly hypoglycaemic the fetus with its increased insulin production is no longer protected by maternal hyperglycaemia and it is possible that some fetuses die *in utero* of hypoglycaemia.

The precise aetiology of congenital malformations is not known. It has been postulated that poor diabetic control at the time of conception and organogenesis (6–8 weeks) may be important. The increased incidence is seen in insulin treated diabetics and rises in those with severe complications.

Pregnant diabetics may be classified into three main groups.

Diabetes presenting during pregnancy

Diabetes presenting in pregnancy may remain permanently or may remit after delivery. (See Table 11.2.)

If glucose tolerance becomes normal after delivery, this is called gestational diabetes. About 15% of our patients fall into this category and in the majority of them the diabetes is apparently 'mild' requiring dietary treatment alone. However the risks to the fetus are, in our experience, just as great as in the insulin treated established diabetic.

Of 25 patients with diabetes diagnosed in pregnancy in 1971–75, six remained diabetic after delivery and 14 had true gestational diabetes, of whom two later became diabetic. Thus eight out of 25 patients (32%) are permanently diabetic within 5 years. It is difficult to know if diabetes would have occurred or been diagnosed so soon without the pregnancy. Some girls do show worsening patterns through successive pregnancies but others have normal glucose tolerance after gestational diabetes in one pregnancy.

Table 11.2 Pregnancy onset 1971–75

	Total	25 (15% of 173)
	Gestational	14 (2 later diabetic)
	Remained diabetic	6 (2 borderline at 2nd GTT)
	Not known	5
Treatment:	Insulin	6
	Diet	19
	Perinatal mortality	0

Established diabetes

Most of these patients are on insulin and a small proportion have minor complications, e.g. mild background retinopathy.

Established diabetes with severe complications (e.g. severe retinopathy, neuropathy or nephropathy)

These patients are rare in our practise; we try to avoid the problem by advising them not to become pregnant. They have a higher incidence of complications during the pregnancy than those in groups 1 and 2. They have also been shown to have a higher incidence of congenital malformations (Pedersen *et al.*, 1964).

DIAGNOSIS OF DIABETES DURING PREGNANCY

Since the risks to the fetus are the same early diagnosis is important. The literature is difficult to interpret since people have used different tests of glucose tolerance and different criteria of abnormality.

We use a standard 2-hour 50 g oral glucose tolerance test and apply the British Diabetic Association criteria as for non-pregnant patients. Random glycosuria may be very common in pregnancy and it is an unreliable indicator

Table 11.3 Indications for GTT in pregnancy

Second fasting specimen glycosuria
First degree family history
Previous babies larger than 4·5 kg
Previous unexplained perinatal deaths
Maternal obesity (more than 20% above ideal weight)
Acute hydramnios
Previous gestational diabetes

119

of possible diabetes. The incidence of diabetes in this group is 2%. If glycosuria is found in a second fasting specimen (produced by voiding the overnight urine in the bladder and collecting a second specimen before breakfast) the incidence of abnormal glucose tolerance rises to 15% (Sutherland *et al.*, 1970). This is thus a better screening test for diabetes than random glycosuria alone. Potential diabetics (see Table 11.3) have a prevalence of diabetes of 6% (Soler and Malins, 1971).

MEDICAL MANAGEMENT OF DIABETES IN PREGNANCY

The aims of treatment are to maintain as near physiological blood sugars as possible without hypoglycaemia. In out-patients this means a blood glucose below 8·5 mmol/l and in-patients below 5 mmol/l.

The majority of patients are on insulin, usually two injections daily in a mixture of soluble and Isophane insulin. Figure 11.1 illustrates the duration and peak effects of these two insulins.

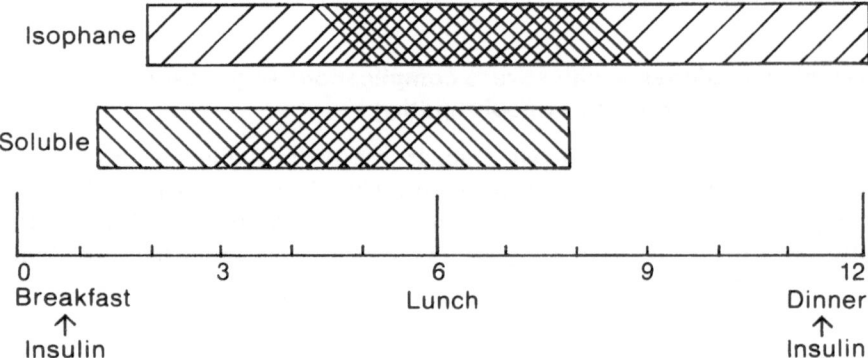

Figure 11.1   Peak effects of soluble and isophane insulins

The patients are seen regularly in a diabetic antenatal clinic by both physicians and obstetricians at the same time. All patients are admitted at 32 weeks and remain in hospital until delivery. On in-patients we do at least twice weekly blood glucose series, before lunch and at 9 p.m. to assess the peak effect of soluble insulin and at 6 p.m. and 6 a.m. for the peak effect of Isophane insulin. The insulin dosages are adjusted frequently if blood glucose is not satisfactory and although we maintain low average blood glucose values symptomatic hypoglycaemia is rare, perhaps because the patients are resting in bed. I think hypoglycaemia (below 3 mmol/l) should be avoided as should wide variations of blood glucose although obviously blood glucose level does vary far more than in normal women. Insulin requirements usually rise by at least 50% especially in the last trimester of pregnancy. Falling insulin requirements in late pregnancy may be an ominous sign particularly if associated with other factors such as falling oestriol levels, placental lactogen and poor fetal growth as shown on ultrasound measurements of biparietal diameter.

ORAL HYPOGLYCAEMIC DRUGS

We do not use oral drugs at any stage of pregnancy. There is no evidence that they are teratogenic so our reluctance to use them in early pregnancy is perhaps emotional. They are certainly contraindicated late in pregnancy as they cross the placenta and may cause severe neonatal hypoglycaemia if administered within 10 days of delivery.

MANAGEMENT OF LABOUR

On the morning of induction breakfast and normal insulin dose are omitted and a continuous infusion of insulin is set up using a motorized pump. Insulin is infused at the rate of 1–2 units per hour and adjusted if necessary to maintain a blood glucose below 7 mmol/l. If delivery is by elective Caesarean section soluble insulin is given 2 hourly according to blood glucose.

After delivery the insulin requirement falls to pre-pregnant levels and we usually commence this dose when glycosuria reappears. Breast feeding does not usually alter the insulin requirements. The patient may require additional dietary carbohydrate to compensate for the losses in breast milk.

OBSTETRIC MANAGEMENT

There is only time to mention briefly the obstetric aspects relevant to these patients. Fetal growth is monitored by serial ultrasound measurements of biparietal diameter. Biochemical estimations of oestriols and placental lactogens are also performed but seem to make little impact on the management at present.

Amniocentesis and measurement of lecithin/sphingomyelin ratios has made a vital difference. All these infants are premature but respiratory distress syndrome is no longer a problem. If the L/S ratio is low then the procedure is repeated a few days later. Dexamethasone is used to induce lecithin production if it is thought imperative to deliver the baby urgently, or if premature labour ensues. Most patients are delivered at $37\frac{1}{2}$ weeks. With the use of fetal monitoring to detect fetal distress vaginal delivery is a safe alternative to elective Caesarean section and this is now the method of choice in primigravidae. 80% of primips now have vaginal delivery at King's although the overall rate is lower. Elective Caesarean section is performed in all women who had previous Caesarean sections and for the usual obstetric indications.

121

RESULTS OF TREATMENT

The average blood glucose value in patients is 4·9 mmol/l (Table 11.4).

Table 11.4 Blood glucose in pregnant diabetics (32–38 weeks)—1973

No. of patients	No. observations	No. blood glucose values		Mean
		> 150 mg/100 ml	> 200 mg/100 ml	
26	940	44 (4·7%)	6 (0·6%)	87 mg/100 ml

Table 11.5 shows the birthweights of infants compared with those 10 years earlier. Although these infants are still approximately 150 g overweight for their gestational age the average birthweight has in fact fallen although the gestational age is slightly greater.

Table 11.5 Infant weights

Years	Number of infants	Average birthweight (g)	Average gestational age (days)
1961–62	88	3282	256
1971–72	76	3329	264
1973	34	3173	262

Perinatal mortality has not only shown a decline but there has been a change in the pattern of causes. Congenital malformation now accounts for a higher proportion of deaths and apparently unexplained stillbirths are now very unusual (Table 11.6).

Table 11.6 Causes of perinatal deaths

Years	Total deliveries	Total perinatal deaths	Obstetric causes	Congenital abnormalities	Diabetic ketosis	Respiratory distress syndrome	Unknown
1961–65	213	24	5	4	1	4	10
1971–75	173	6	1	3	1	0	1

There is an increased perinatal morbidity in infants of diabetic mothers. Symptomatic hypoglycaemia is unusual but chemical hypoglycaemia occurs in about 17% of babies. Early feeding is the rule and this is supplemented with intravenous glucose infusion if hypoglycaemia persists. Hyperbilirubinaemia occurs in a similar number of babies; respiratory distress is extremely unusual, but tachypnoea may occur. There is an increased incidence of congenital malformation in these infants. In the last 5 years at King's the incidence was 7·5% (see Table 11.7) and this seems to be an increase over the previous 10 years. A similar increase has been reported from Birmingham and it is difficult to know the significance of this. Teratogenic effects of insulin in animals have been reported (Landauer, 1972). It may be significant that the higher incidence of congenital malformations is only seen in patients on insulin (Soler *et al.*, 1976).

Table 11.7 Congenital malformations in infants of diabetic mothers 1961–1975

1961–65	4/213	1 Multiple		d.
		1 CHD		d.
		1 Neural canal		d.
		1 Absent kidneys		d.
1966–70	3/176	2 CHD + hemivertebrae	2	d.
		1 Imperforate anus		d.
1971–75	13/173	4 CHD	2	d.
		2 Neural canal	1	d.
		2 Cleft palate/harelip		
		1 CHD		
		2 Skeletal (1 sacral agenesis)		
		1 Choanal atresia	(late death)	
		1 Exomphalos		d.

Despite the continued improvement in results we have no grounds for complacency. Although most perinatal deaths now seem to be apparently unavoidable in the present state of knowledge, we have in the last year at King's College Hospital had two patients experience intrauterine deaths in the 38th week of pregnancy, one an established diabetic with mild pre-eclampsia, the other a gestational diabetic on diet only. In neither of these patients was there any warning that the fetus was in danger. These tragedies emphasize the need for continued vigilance in caring for these patients, and further research to try to elucidate the many problems that we do not yet understand.

References

Baird, J. D. and Farquhar, J. W. (1962). Insulin-secreting capacity in newborn infants of normal and diabetic women. *Lancet*, **i**, 71

de Gasparo, and Hoet, J. J. (1971). Diabetes. *Proceedings of 7th International Diabetes Conference*, p. 667

Landauer, W. (1972). Is insulin a teratogen? *Teratology*, **5**, 129

Soler, N. G. and Malins, J. M. (1971). Indications for oral glucose-tolerance tests during pregnancy. *Lancet*, **ii**, 724

Soler, N. G., Walsh, C. H. and Malins, J. M. (1976). Studies in whole body potassium and whole body nitrogen in newly diagnosed diabetics. *Q. J. Med.*, **45**, 295

Sutherland, H. W., Stowers, J. M. and McKenzie, C. (1970). Simplifying the clinical problem of glycosuria in pregnancy. *Lancet*, **i**, 1069

General Reading

Essex, N. (1976). Diabetes and pregnancy. *Br. J. Hosp. Med.*, **15**, 333

Sutherland, H. W. and Stowers, J. M. (1975). *Carbohydrate Metabolism in Pregnancy and the Newborn*. (Edinburgh: Churchill-Livingstone)

Part 4
Drugs and the Fetus

12
Maternal Drug Therapy and Enzyme Induction in the Fetus and Newborn

D. S. DAVIES and A. R. BOOBIS*

INTRODUCTION

Most drugs are lipid soluble at physiological pH. This aids absorption from the gastrointestinal tract and penetration of body membranes but greatly hinders excretion in urine or bile. The intensity and duration of pharmacological action of a lipid soluble drug are thus largely governed by the rate at which it is converted to more polar, often inactive, metabolites. Drug metabolism may be thought of as occurring in two phases (Williams, 1959); in phase I functional chemical groups may be changed, e.g. the conversion of an alcohol to an aldehyde or new ones introduced, e.g. hydroxylation of aromatic rings. Phase II involves synthetic reactions, those in which functional groups are conjugated with glucuronate, sulphate and a variety of other compounds derived from carbohydrate or amino acid metabolism.

Many lipid soluble drugs are metabolized by phase I oxidative reactions which are catalysed by enzyme systems found mainly in hepatic endoplasmic reticulum. These enzymes, known as mixed function oxidases, consist of NADPH-cytochrome c reductase coupled to carbon monoxide sensitive hemoproteins, generally known as cytochromes P-450. Drug substrates combine with oxidized cytochrome P-450 to form complexes which are reduced by NADPH-cytochrome c reductase. The reduced complex interacts with molecular oxygen which is then 'activated' by the transfer of a second electron via NADPH-cytochrome c reductase and then re-arranges to give oxidized drug, cytochrome P-450, and water.

---

* Recipient of MRC Training Fellowship.

It has been known since the work of Remmer (1962) and Conney and Burns (1962) in the early 1960s that the chronic administration of certain drugs and other chemicals can increase the activity of some drug metabolizing enzymes, particularly the cytochrome P-450 dependent mixed function oxidases. More than 200 drugs and other chemicals are now known to induce drug metabolism in laboratory animals and in man resulting in diminished therapeutic response in some cases and increased toxicity in others (Conney, 1967). It was therefore of considerable importance to determine:

(a) if the fetal liver metabolized drugs
(b) was this drug metabolizing ability, if it existed, induced by the administration of drugs to the mother.

DRUG METABOLISM IN THE FETUS AND NEWBORN

Early studies suggested that fetal and newborn laboratory animals were unable to oxidize many drugs (Jondorf et al., 1958; Fouts and Adamson, 1959; Netter, 1975). Recent studies, utilizing sensitive analytical methods, have shown the presence of cytochrome P-450 in fetal livers from animals during the final third period of pregnancy (Gillette et al., 1973; Welch et al., 1972). However, enzyme activities were variable and were only about 1% of those found in livers obtained from the mothers.

Because of the results obtained in laboratory animals it had been assumed that fetal and newborn man would have little or no ability to metabolize drugs, especially by oxidative reactions. This was, to some extent, supported by clinical observations and newborn infants appeared to be more sensitive to the action of some drugs. However, in the early 1970s, it was shown that cytochrome P-450 is present in human fetal liver (Yaffe

Table 12.1 Maximal velocities (Vm) for the N-demethylation of ethylmorphine by fetal and adult human liver microsomal enzymes

	Gestational age (weeks)	Vm (nmol/mg/min)
Fetus	14 (3)	1·33
	25 (1)	2·47
	35 (1)	3·50
Adult (10)	—	5·20

et al., 1970) as early as the 12th week of gestation (Pelkonen, 1973) and increases to approximately 30% of the adult value in the 35th week of gestation (Thorgeirsson, 1971). A number of model substrates are metabolized by human fetal liver enzymes including aminopyrine, chlorpromazine, aniline, N-methylaniline and ethylmorphine (Yaffe et al., 1970; Thorgeirsson,

1971; Pelkonen et al., 1971; Rane and Ackerman, 1971). Benzo-(a)-pyrene hydroxylase is detectable in the 6th week of gestation (Pelkonen, 1973). Activities are low early in pregnancy but in the case of ethylmorphine N-demethylase (Thorgeirsson, 1971) maximal velocities are 66% of adult value at a gestational age of 35 weeks (Table 12.1).

It came as no surprise, therefore, to find that the newborn infant, unlike laboratory animals, is well able to metabolize a variety of drugs and other chemicals (Horning et al., 1975). Rates of in vivo metabolism of drugs have been compared in newborn infants and adults, usually their mothers. The mean plasma half-life of amylobarbitone was about twice as long in newborn infants as in their mothers (Krauer et al., 1973) (Table 12.2). Plasma half-lives of antipyrine (Murdock et al., 1975) given intravenously to 21

Table 12.2 Plasma half-lives of drugs in newborn and adult humans

	Plasma half-life (h)	
Drug	Newborn	Adult
Antipyrine	58·6 (21)	10·4 (20)
Amylobarbitone	37·8 (8)	20·0 (9)
Phenytoin	17·4 (5)	22·2 (18)

infants on their first day of life averaged 58·6 h as compared to 10·4 h in a group of 20 unrelated adults. By day 4 the mean half-life for antipyrine had fallen to 20·8 h (Table 12.2).

However, newborn infants of epileptic mothers on long-term treatment with phenytoin appeared to metabolize the drug as rapidly as adults (Rane et al., 1974) (Table 12.2). It was suggested that transplacentally transferred phenytoin may induce the drug oxidizing enzymes before birth.

TRANSPLACENTAL ENZYME INDUCTION IN THE FETUS AND NEWBORN

Drugs cross the placenta by a number of ways including pinocytosis and in a few instances by facilitative or active transport systems. However, most drugs simply diffuse across the placenta and this is largely governed by the physico-chemical properties of the drug and the physiological properties of the placental barrier. Numerous studies have shown that the rate of transport of most drugs across the placenta is proportional to the fraction of unbound, unionized drug in maternal plasma and to the lipid solubility of the unionized form of the drug (Mirkin, 1975). Since most enzyme inducing agents are lipid soluble at physiological pH they might be expected to readily cross the placenta but would they induce fetal drug metabolizing enzymes?

Induction of conjugating enzymes

In one of the earliest attempts to induce drug-metabolizing enzymes in fetal and newborn animals, Inscoe and Axelrod (1960) found that the administration of benzo-(a)-pyrene, a potent inducing agent, to pregnant rats did not increase fetal hepatic glucuronyl transferase activity. However, there was induction of the transferase in maternal and neonatal livers. The latter observation led to the suggestion that enzyme inducing agents administered to the mother may be of value in lowering the incidence and severity of neonatal jaundice.

Numerous studies have shown that the elimination of bilirubin is facilitated and serum-bilirubin concentrations decreased in neonatal infants born to mothers receiving phenobarbitone during pregnancy (Trolle, 1968; Maurer *et al.*, 1968). This has generally been assumed to be due to an increase in glucuronyl transferase activity in the neonatal liver. However, in recent studies (Orme *et al.*, 1974) it was found that although antipyrine, like phenobarbitone, lowers total serum-bilirubin in patients with Gilbert's syndrome only the former drug increases the activity of hepatic bilirubin glucuronyl transferase in rats (Table 12.3). Phenobarbitone administration

Table 12.3 Effect of phenobarbitone and antipyrine on bilirubin conjugation by rat liver microsomes

Treatment (mmol/kg/24 h)	Vmax (nmol/30 min/mg)	Km (µmol/l)
None	$14 \cdot 47 \pm 1 \cdot 48$	$67 \cdot 7 \pm 10 \cdot 5$
Antipyrine (1·27)	$25 \cdot 03 \pm 4 \cdot 28$	$85 \cdot 6 \pm 20 \cdot 0$
Phenobarbitone (0·34)	$14 \cdot 93 \pm 0 \cdot 49$	$62 \cdot 3 \pm 5 \cdot 9$

has been shown to increase liver blood flow (Ohnhaus *et al.*, 1974), bile flow (Klaasen and Plaa, 1968) and hepatic binding proteins (Reyes *et al.*, 1969) all of which may contribute to the lowering of total serum-bilirubin. Recently, an increased rate of transfer of bilirubin from liver to bile has been implicated in the stimulatory effects of inducers on bilirubin clearance in the neonate (Klaasen, 1976).

It was not necessarily valid, therefore, to conclude that lowered serum-bilirubin concentrations in newborn infants of mothers treated with phenobarbitone are the result of enzyme induction in the neonatal liver.

Induction of cytochrome P-450 dependent mixed-function oxidases

Initial studies showed that pretreatment of pregnant rabbits with phenobarbitone did not increase the rate of oxidation of hexobarbitone by fetal liver enzymes as late as 4 days before term (Hart *et al.*, 1962). At term and in the newborn rabbit there were considerable increases in hexobarbitone hydroxylase activities (Table 12.4). Similar results have been obtained in other studies utilizing a variety of inducing agents and drug substrates,

Table 12.4 **Effects of maternal administration of phenobarbitone on hexo-barbitone* metabolism by fetal and newborn rabbit liver**

	Fetus		Newborn
	Pre-term (4 days)	Term	
Control	0 (7)	0 (7)	0·08 ± 0·18 (6)
Treated†	0 (6)	0·96 ± 0·98 (10)	1·55 ± 0·69 (10)

* μmol/g/h
† 15 mg/kg/day for 4 days

although recently induction of benzo-(a)-pyrene hydroxylase activity to 50% of adult levels has been shown in the rabbit at 5 days before term (Atlas *et al.*, 1977). The difficulty of inducing drug metabolizing enzymes transplacentally was confirmed by Welch and his colleagues (1972) who found that a 20-fold greater dose of benzo-(a)-pyrene was required to stimulate the hydroxylation of aromatic hydrocarbons by fetal liver than was needed for the mother. The limited information available from studies in man support the view that transplacental enzyme induction does not readily occur. Pelkonen and colleagues (Pelkonen *et al.*, 1972) found that whereas maternal cigarette smoking stimulated benzo-(a)-pyrene metabolism by the placenta it had no effect on the metabolism of the same substrate by the fetal liver. The N-demethylation of N-methylaniline was not increased in either the placenta or fetal liver obtained from cigarette smokers (Table 12.5). The same

Table 12.5 **Effects of cigarette smoking* on 3, 4-benzpyrene (BP) hydroxylase and N-methyl-aniline (MA) demethylase in fetal liver and placenta**

Mothers	BP hydroxylase (nmol/g/h)		MA demethylase (μmol/g/h)	
	Liver	Placenta	Liver	Placenta
Smokers (9)	0·21 ± 0·04	0·08 ± 0·01	0·73 ± 0·09	0·10 ± 0·05
Non-smokers (9)	0·22 ± 0·06	<0·02	0·77 ± 0·23	0·10 ± 0·04

* Mean 13·3/day

workers (Pelkonen *et al.*, 1973) were unable to demonstrate statistically significant increases in the metabolism of chlorpromazine or *p*-nitrobenzoic acid by fetal livers obtained from mothers pretreated with phenobarbitone (100 mg/day) for 7–25 days (Table 12.6).

Rates of elimination of drugs by newborn infants of mothers receiving drugs during pregnancy confirm that transplacental enzyme induction is not readily achieved with the usual inducing agents. Half-lives of antipyrine in newborn infants of mothers receiving barbiturates were within the normal

Table 12.6 Effect of maternal administration of phenobarbitone on the metabolism of chlorpromazine (CPZ) and P-nitrobenzoic acid (PNA) by human fetal liver

	Phenobarbitone (100 mg/day)	Fetal weight (g)	CPZ (μmol/g/h)	PNA (μmol/g/h)
Controls (11)	—	146 ± 62	0·14 ± 0·02	0·07 ± 0·02
Treated (8)	7–15 days	136 ± 60	0·17 ± 0·02	0·10 ± 0·02

range and were influenced more by the clinical state of the child than the drug intake of the mother. Similarly, plasma half-lives of transplacentally transferred amylobarbitone were similar in newborn infants whether the mothers had received a single dose immediately before delivery or multiple inducing doses during the pregnancy (Draffan *et al.*, 1976). Nor did prior treatment with phenobarbitone have any significant effect on plasma half-lives of amylobarbitone in newborn infants (Figure 12.1).

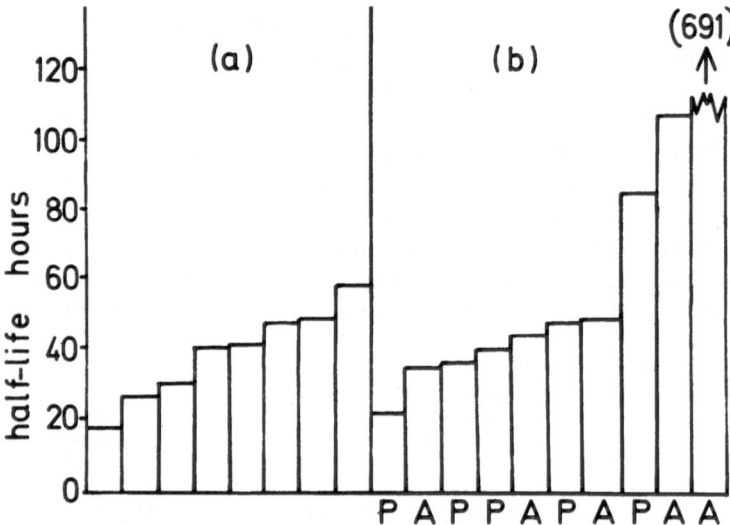

Figure 12.1 Plasma half-lives of amylobarbitone.
(a) in newborn infants whose mothers had received a single dose of amylobarbitone during labour;
(b) in newborn infants whose mothers had also received prolonged treatment with phenobarbitone (P) or amylobarbitone (A).
(Reproduced from *Clinical Pharmacology and Therapeutics*)

Thus man is similar to laboratory animals in that little or no induction of fetal liver enzymes is achieved with inducing agents such as barbiturates given in doses which do increase enzyme activities in the maternal liver. However, whereas the newborn of laboratory animals show considerable enzyme induction following pretreatment of their mothers this does not happen in man.

Numerous explanations have been offered for the failure to induce fetal liver enzymes ranging from an inability to respond to the stimulus to lack of sufficiently high concentrations of the inducing agent in the fetal liver. It is true that most inducing agents are given orally or, in laboratory animals, intraperitoneally thus presenting high concentrations to the maternal liver at the 'first pass'. The achievement of similar concentrations in the fetal liver may be limited by the maternal toxicity of the inducing agent. However, this pharmacokinetic explanation does not explain why it is possible to induce rabbit fetal livers late but not early in pregnancy (Hart *et al.*, 1962). Thus an inability to respond to the inducing agent appears to be the more likely explanation for the lack of induction early in pregnancy. Recent studies, however, have shown that with the right inducing agent positive results can be achieved early in pregnancy.

The herbicide contaminant 2, 3, 7, 8-tetrachlorodibenzo-*p*-dioxin (TCDD) (it recently polluted the Italian town of Seveso) given to rats in a single dose of $2·5\,\mu g/kg$ on day 17 of gestation produced considerable induction of aryl hydrocarbon hydroxylase activity in maternal and fetal livers (Berry *et al.*, 1976). Thus the lack of response to some of the other agents was not due to the absence of appropriate structural and/or regulatory genes required for the expression of enzyme induction during fetal life. Although attempts to show induction of human fetal liver enzymes *in vivo* have failed, it has recently been shown that human fetal liver cultures are inducible *in vitro* (Pelkonen *et al.*, 1975). Thus human fetal liver also possesses the necessary genes to respond to hydrocarbon inducers.

TCDD and many polycyclic hydrocarbons such as benzo-(a)-pyrene interact with a common 'induction receptor' in the cell cytosol. Phenobarbitone and other similar inducers do not interact with this receptor and most probably interact with a different receptor. The affinity of the hydrocarbon receptor is several thousand times higher for TCDD than for compounds such as benzo-(a)-pyrene. This mechanism of induction provides several possible explanations for the conflicting results described above. The nature of the receptor may change during development so that its affinity for compounds other than TCDD increases. Alternatively, the number of 'induction receptors' may increase with fetal age. A third possibility is that the acceptor site for the receptor on the DNA alters with development so that a wider variety of compounds can produce a response in more mature fetuses. Fetal induction, therefore, may be a true differentiation phenomenon and evidence to this effect has been obtained (Atlas *et al.*, 1977). A likely explanation for the lack of response of the fetus to phenobarbitone is that the receptor for this compound probably does not develop until late on in pregnancy. Lack of any induction in the human fetus *in vivo* could be due to repression of receptor formation or the fact that for ethical reasons it is not possible to study the fetal response to appropriate inducers such as TCDD in man.

THE ROLE OF DRUG METABOLISM BY FETAL TISSUE ENZYMES

The presence of drug metabolizing enzymes in the human fetus raised the possibility that they might have a role in limiting exposure of the fetus to drugs and other environmental chemicals. However, as has been pointed out by Gillette and Stripp (1975), this would only be of value if the fetal liver were able to extract most of the drug at the 'first pass' before it enters the fetal hepatic vein. The 'first pass' effect occurs with relatively few drugs in adults and is unlikely to be of more importance in the fetus where enzyme activities are lower. Thus fetal hepatic enzymes do not appear to have a significant role in protecting the fetus against lipid-soluble chemicals. However, these enzymes may play a significant role in the fetotoxicities of a variety of chemicals.

Studies during the past few years have shown that cytochrome P-450 enzyme systems in liver of adult animals can convert chemically inactive molecules to reactive arylating or alkylating metabolites which may bind covalently to tissue macromolecules thereby causing toxicity or carcinogenicity (Gillette *et al.*, 1974). The human fetus is better able to carry out these reactions than the fetuses of most laboratory animals and this should be borne in mind when extrapolating teratogenic data obtained in animals to man.

There is considerable interest currently in the possible teratogenic effects of the anti-epileptic drug phenytoin (e.g. see Chapter 10). Preliminary studies by Blake and Fallinger (1976) suggest that a chemically reactive epoxide of

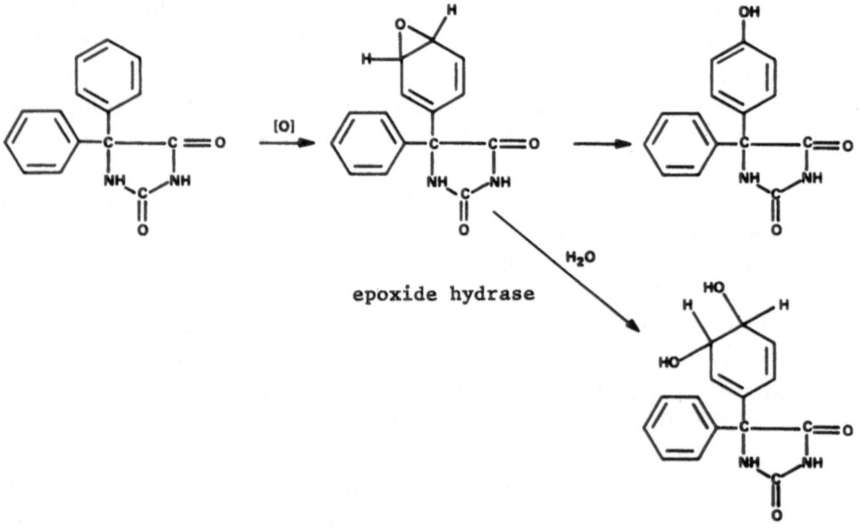

Figure 12.2 Aromatic hydroxylation of phenytoin: formation of an epoxide and its conversion to a phenol or dihydrodiol

phenytoin generated by the cytochrome P-450 enzyme system may be involved in the drug's teratogenic effects. Epoxides generated by the P-450 system can undergo a variety of fates including conversion to a dihydrodiol mediated by the enzyme epoxide hydrase (Figure 12.2). Blake and Fallinger found that treatment of pregnant mice with phenytoin and a potent inhibitor of epoxide hydrase (trichloropropene oxide) significantly increased the incidence of orofacial anomalies in the offspring, suggesting that removal of the protective pathway by inhibition of the hydrase allowed more of the chemically reactive epoxide to bind covalently to macromolecules and cause toxicity. Further studies are needed to confirm these findings but they serve to emphasize the importance not only of studying the development of the P-450 enzymes in the human fetus but also other enzyme systems such as epoxide hydrase and the various transferases which have a protective role in the cell. In addition it is important to identify drugs and chemicals in the environment which may endanger the fetus by selectively inducing fetal P-450 systems or by inhibiting protective pathways.

References

Atlas, S. A., Boobis, A. R., Thorgeirsson, S. S. and Nebert, D. W. (1977). Ontogenetic expression of polycyclic aromatic compound-inducible monooxygenase activities and forms of cytochrome P-450 in the rabbit. Evidence for temporal control and organ specificity of two genetic regulatory systems. *J. Biol. Chem.* (In press)

Berry, D. L., Zachariah, P. K., Namkung, M. J. and Jachau, M. R. (1976). Transplacental induction of carcinogen-hydroxylating systems with 2, 3, 7, 8-tetrachlorodibenzo-*p*-dioxin. *Toxicol. Appl. Pharmacol.*, **36**, 569

Blake, D. A. and Fallinger, C. (1976). Embryopathic interaction of phenytoin and trichloropropene oxide in mice. *Teratology*, **13**, 17a

Conney, A. H. (1967). Pharmacological implications of microsomal enzyme induction. *Pharmacol. Rev.*, **19**, 317

Conney, A. H. and Burns, B. B. (1962). Factors influencing drug metabolism. *Arch. Pharmacol.*, **1**, 31

Draffan, G. H., Dollery, C. T., Davies, D. S., Krauer, B., Williams, F. M., Clare, R. A., Trudinger, B. J., Darling, M., Sertel, H. and Hawkins, D. F. (1976). Maternal and neonatal elimination of amobarbital after treatment of the mother with barbiturates during late pregnancy. *Clin. Pharmacol. Ther.*, **19**, 271

Fouts, J. R. and Adamson, R. H. (1959). Drug metabolism in newborn rabbits. *Science*, **129**, 897

Gillette, J. R. and Stripp, B. (1975). Pre- and postnatal enzyme capacity for drug metabolite production. *Fed. Proc.*, **34**, 172

Gillette, J. R., Menard, R. H. and Stripp, B. (1973). *Clin. Pharmacol. Ther.*, **14**, 680

Gillette, J. R. Mitchell, J. R. and Brodie, B. B. (1974). Biochemical basis for drug toxicity. *Ann. Rev. Pharmacol.*, **14**, 271

Hart, L. G., Adamson, R. H., Dixon, R. L. and Fouts, J. R. (1962). Stimulation of hepatic microsomal drug metabolism in the newborn and foetal rabbit. *J. Pharmac. Exp. Ther.*, **137**, 103

Horning, M. G., Butler, C. M., Nowlin, J. and Hill, R. M. (1975). Drug metabolism in human neonate. *Life Sci.*, **16**, 651

Inscoe, J. K. and Axelrod, J. (1960). Some factors effecting glucuronide formation *in vitro*. *J. Pharmacol. Exp. Ther.*, **129**, 128

Jondorf, W. R., Maickel, R. P. and Brodie, B. B. (1958). Inability of newborn mice and guinea pigs to metabolize drugs. *Biochem. Pharmacol.*, **1**, 352

Klaassen, C. D. (1976). Effect of microsomal enzyme inducers on the biliary excretion of an exogenous load of bilirubin in newborn rats. *Proc. Soc. Exp. Biol. Med.*, **153**, 370

Klaassen, C. D. and Plaa, G. L. (1968). Studies on the mechanics of phenobarbital enhanced sulfobromophthalein disappearance. *J. Lab. Clin. Med.*, **81**, 829

Krauer, B., Draffan, G. H., Williams, F. M., Clare, R. A., Dollery, C. T. and Hawkins, D. F. (1973). Elimination kinetics of amobarbital in mothers and newborn infants. *Clin. Pharmacol. Ther.*, **14**, 442

Maurer, H. M., Wolff, J. A., Poppers, P. J., Finster, M., Pantuck, E., Kuntzman, R. and Conney, A. H. (1968). Reduction in concentration of total serum-bilirubin in offspring of women treated with phenobarbitone during pregnancy. *Lancet*, **ii**, 122

Mirkin, B. L. (1975). Placental transfer, fetal localization and neonatal disposition of drugs. *Anesthesiology*, **43**, 156

Murdock, A. I., Thorgeirsson, S. S., Rossiger, H. and Davies, D. S. (1975). Serial measurements of plasma half-lives and urinary excretion of antipyrine in low birthweight infants. *Biol. Neonate*, **27**, 289

Netter, K. (1975). Developmental aspects of drug metabolism. *Proceedings of the 6th International Congress of Pharmacology*, **6**, 3

Ohnhaus, E. E., Thorgeirsson, S. S., Davies, D. S. and Breckenridge, A. M. (1971). Changes in liver blood flow during enzyme induction. *Biochem. Pharmacol.*, **20**, 861

Orme, M. L'E., Davies, L. and Breckenridge, A. M. (1974). Increased glucuronidation of bilirubin in man and rat by administration of antipyrine (phenazone). *Clin. Sci. Mol. Med.*, **46**, 511

Pelkonen, O. (1973). Studies on drug metabolizing enzymes in the human fetus. PhD Thesis, University of Oulu, Finland

Pelkonen, O., Arvela, P. and Karki, N. T. (1971). 3, 4-Benzpyrene and *N*-methylaniline metabolizing enzymes in the immature human foetus and placenta. *Acta Pharmacol. Toxicol.*, **30**, 385

Pelkonen, O., Jouppila, P. and Karki, N. T. (1972). Effect of maternal cigarette smoking on 3, 4-benzpyrene and *N*-methylaniline metabolism in human fetal liver and placenta. *Toxicol. Appl. Pharmacol.*, **23**, 399

Pelkonen, O., Jouppila, P. and Karki, N. T. (1973). Attempts to induce drug metabolism in human fetal liver and placenta by the administration of phenobarbital to mothers. *Arch. Int. Pharmacodyn. Ther.*, **202**, 288

Pelkonen, O., Korhonen, P., Jouppila, P. and Karki, N. T. (1975). *Life Sci.*, **16**, 1403

Pelkonen, O., Vorne, M., Jouppila, P. and Karki, N. T. (1971). Metabolism of chlorpromazine and *p*-nitrobenzoic acid in the liver, intestine and kidney of the human foetus. *Acta Pharmacol. Toxicol.*, **29**, 294

Rane, A. and Ackerman, E. (1971). Metabolism of ethylmorphine and aniline in human foetal liver. *Clin. Pharmacol. Ther.*, **13**, 663

Rane, A., Garle, M., Bora, O. and Sjoqvist, F. (1974). Plasma disappearance of transplacentally transferred diphenylhydantoin in the newborn studied by mass fragmentography. *Clin. Pharmacol. Ther.*, **15**, 39

Remmer, H. (1962). Drugs as activators of drug enzymes. In: Metabolic factors controlling duration of drug actions. *Proceedings 1st International Pharmacology Meeting*, Vol. 6, B. B. Brodie and E. G. Erdos (eds.), p. 235 (New York: Macmillan)

Reyes, H., Levi, A. J., Gatmaitan, Z. and Arias, I. M. (1969). Organic anion-binding protein in rat liver: drug induction and its physiological consequence. *Proc. Nat. Acad. Sci. U.S.A.*, **64**, 168

Thorgeirsson, S. S. (1971). Mechanism of hepatic drug oxidation and its relationship to individual differences in rates of oxidation in man. PhD Thesis, University of London

Trolle, E. (1968). Decrease of total serum-bilirubin concentration in newborn infants after phenobarbitone treatment. *Lancet*, **ii**, 705

Welch, R. M. Gommi, B., Alvarez, A. P. and Conney, A. H. (1972). Effect of enzyme induction in the metabolism of benzo-(a)-pyrene and 3'-methyl-4-monomethylaminoazobenzene in the pregnant and fetal rat. *Cancer Res.*, **32**, 973

Williams, R. T. (1959). *Detoxication Mechanisms*, 2nd Ed. (London: Chapman and Hall)

Yaffe, S. J., Rane, A., Sjoqvist, F., Boreus, L.-O. and Orrenuis, S. (1970). The presence of a mono-oxygenase system in human foetal liver microsomes. *Life Sci.*, **9**, 1189

Discussion

Herxheimer: Are there any substances that the pregnant woman is likely to encounter which might have a similar effect to TCDD? Are there any therapeutic substances which might have a similar effect?

Davies: I do not think there are any drugs with a similar action but polychlorinated biphenyls appear very widely in the environment and may have similar effects. I think the answer is that pregnant women could be so exposed from the environment.

Herxheimer: So women who are employed working with these chemicals would be a risk group who ought to be examined?

Davies: I do not want to raise scares but women working in that sort of environment might well be at risk.

Herxheimer: What about the insecticides used in the treatment for pediculosis for example? Substances such as malathion.

Davies: These substances are not related to TCDD but they should probably be looked at. I should put this in proportion however by saying that TCDD is by far the most powerful compound with this action.

Lewis: What do you think the tetiological advantage to the fetus is of having all these hepatic enzymes switched off while it remains *in utero*?

Davies: Well I suppose some of these toxic effects which I described do arise from having these enzymes switched on *in utero* so perhaps there is an advantage of the fetus in not having this activity. I think one of the problems in interpreting these data is the number of competitive substances which are present in the fetus and newborn which disguise the enzyme activity. For example steroids are alternative substrates for these enzymes and do compete. These competitive substances might explain some of the lower activity seen *in vivo* but it would not explain the low level of activity seen in *in vitro* experiments.

Lewis: This seems to suggest, doesn't it, that there are some endogenous substances which the fetus is better off not hydroxylating so that they become water soluble and are retained within the fetus.

Davies: That is a possibility that was canvassed some years ago but I understand now that the consensus is that hydroxylated compounds would not be retained in the fetus; they would be eliminated.

Beilin: Is anything known about the effects of drugs of addiction in this regard, opiates, etc.?

Davies: It is reported that alcohol will increase bilirubin conjugation. But again the evidence is from *in vivo* bilirubin levels so this could be due not directly to enzyme

138

induction but to other effects. Indeed, I understand alcohol has been used therapeutically in the United States to lower newborn bilirubin levels. Heroin is an inducing agent. Many of these compounds which are oxidized in the liver and which are lipid soluble are in fact inducing agents. However, they are not in the same class as TCDD.

13
Maternal Drug Therapy and Neonatal Jaundice*

LOUISE A. FRIEDMAN and P. J. LEWIS

INTRODUCTION

Jaundice in the immediate neonatal period is common. The underlying cause of this 'physiological jaundice' is the low capacity of the neonatal liver to conjugate bilirubin to bilirubin glucuronide, the polar conjugate of bilirubin which is excreted in the bile. Other causes of jaundice may be superimposed on this neonatal predisposition (Zuelzer and Brown, 1961). The ability of the neonatal liver to conjugate bilirubin increases rapidly after birth and neonatal jaundice is normally transient. Nevertheless, it may be of serious consequence if the level of bilirubin in the serum is high enough for long enough to precipitate kernicterus or bilirubin encephalopathy of the newborn.

There is some indication that the incidence and severity of neonatal jaundice has increased in recent years (Ghosh and Hudson, 1972; Campbell *et al.*, 1975) and this puts more infants at risk of kernicterus. The factors associated with this increase are not entirely clear; maternal drug therapy has been implicated (Ghosh and Hudson, 1972; Chalmers *et al.*, 1975). This paper reviews the evidence that such an increase in neonatal jaundice has occurred; discusses it in relation to drug therapy and reports some observations on the effect of drugs on the metabolism of bilirubin.

HAS THE INCIDENCE OF NEONATAL JAUNDICE INCREASED?

There have been several suggestions in the literature that an increase in the incidence of neonatal jaundice has occurred in recent years. Attempts have been made to relate this phenomenon to changes in obstetric practice. However,

* This study was supported by the Wellcome Trust.

141

if the literature is examined critically it is difficult to find convincing evidence that an increase in the incidence of neonatal jaundice has actually occurred. There is some doubt that a real phenomenon is being investigated.

Serial studies of incidence

Among the many papers referring to the increasing incidence of neonatal jaundice, only two actually site serial figures of incidence in support of their claims. Sims and Neligan (1975) merely state that the incidence in neonates of a serum bilirubin level of 15 mg/100 ml or over rose from 2·2% in the first 3 months of 1973 to 5·5% in 1974. Campbell *et al.*, (1975) reported a 5-year retrospective analysis of the incidence of neonatal jaundice at Queen Charlotte's Hospital over the period 1969–73. They documented a sharp increase in the incidence of serum bilirubin levels over 12 mg/100 ml in 1972. Their sample excluded babies with rhesus isoimmunization and the percentage incidence of neonates with serum bilirubin levels over 12 mg/100 ml was 6·2, 7·1, 8·1, 12·1 and 15·5 respectively in the years 1969–73.

In view of the paucity of serial studies on the incidence of neonatal jaundice we decided to carry out a retrospective survey on serum bilirubin measurements made at Queen Charlotte's Hospital for the period 1971–6. Since the essential question is whether normal neonates now have an increasing tendency to become jaundiced, the study population was selected to omit all cases of multiple birth, rhesus isoimmunization, ABO incompatibility and G6PD deficiency. Also excluded were all babies who did not remain in the hospital for at least 7 days after delivery, since it was reasoned that infants discharged earlier might develop jaundice at home on the 3rd or 4th day after birth and this would not be recorded in the hospital records. The monthly incidence of significant jaundice as determined in this survey is shown in Figure 13.1. It is apparent that the overall incidence of neonatal jaundice did increase somewhat in 1971 but it has remained fairly constant thereafter with little seasonal bias.

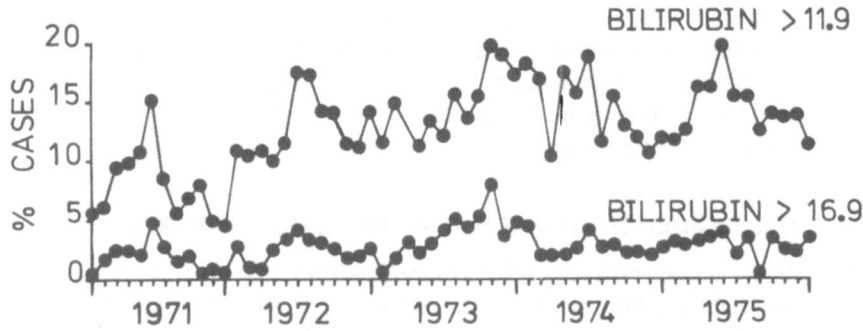

Figure 13.1 Monthly incidence of elevated serum bilirubin concentrations in neonates born at Queen Charlotte's Hospital 1971–5

Jaundice rates

Another possible way of deciding if any increase in neonatal jaundice has occurred in recent years is to gather information on the incidence of neonatal jaundice from the literature. If any change in obstetric practice has affected neonatal bilirubin levels, then early reports should show a different incidence of jaundice. Unfortunately there are few figures in the literature which can be used to establish a normal incidence for neonatal jaundice, especially for the period before the wide adoption of oxytocin induction of labour.

One such early study is that of Billing *et al.* (1954). In this report 49 neonates were selected according to body weight, a preponderance of low birthweight infants being studied. A clear relationship of low birthweight and jaundice was shown. Of interest from the present point of view is that no babies studied with a birthweight over 2·5 kg had a serum bilirubin exceeding 12 mg/100 ml in the first week after birth. By contrast, in our recent large retrospective study we gathered data on 2376 infants weighing between 2·5 and 3·0 kg at birth. 17% of this group had a serum bilirubin greater than 12 mg/100 ml.

Table 13.1 Incidence of neonatal serum bilirubin concentrations over stated figure in various published series

Reference	*% Incidence of bilirubin level* (mg/100 ml)			
	>10	>12	>17	*Total sample*
Trolle, 1968	22·6	15·8	2·9	1469
British Births, 1970, 1975	2·6	—	—	16077
Ghosh and Hudson, 1972	—	12·1	—	197
Dahms *et al.*, 1973	21	—	—	199
Beazley and Alderman, 1975	—	8·4	—	1353
Chalmers *et al.*, 1975	9·2	—	—	10591
Campbell *et al.*, 1975	—	9·8	2·4	18331
Thomas, 1976	16·3	—	1·3	239
This survey	—	12·9	2·7	12543

Other incidence figures in the literature are quoted in Table 13.1. The study populations in each of these publications were chosen in different ways and studied with greater or lesser care. Nevertheless, with the exception of the *British Births Survey 1970* (1975) the incidence of neonatal jaundice is remarkably similar in all these surveys. The low incidence of jaundice quoted in the British Births survey is probably due to the low proportion of babies in this population survey who had a measurement of serum bilirubin. Only 26% of all those reported to be clinically jaundiced had such a measurement. If it were to be assumed that all the clinically jaundiced babies had a similar range of serum bilirubin then the actual incidence of serum bilirubin over

10 mg/100 ml might rise towards 10%, very much more in line with the other series quoted.

It is clear from these figures that the evidence for an increased incidence in neonatal jaundice is rather weak. The variations seen in different studies and at different times may be largely due to the variations in the practice of the paediatrician who decides to measure the serum bilirubin of the baby. Comparison of these epidemiological surveys assumes that this index of suspicion or mere clinical curiosity remains constant over the time investigated. With the appearance of literature linking jaundice with modern obstetric practice it is almost inevitable that the paediatric residents' index of suspicion will drop and an inevitable consequence of this will be an increase in the number of serum bilirubins measured and hence in the incidence of significantly elevated bilirubin levels. It has been demonstrated long ago that the clinical appearance of jaundice in neonates is a poor predictor of serum bilirubin concentration (Davidson et al., 1941) and this is probably a major confounding factor in most reports.

An international survey on the incidence of neonatal jaundice

In order to determine whether any increase in neonatal jaundice has been noted by paediatricians in other centres, a postal survey was undertaken of members of The American Pediatric Society and the European Society for Paediatric Research. The questionnaire sent asked whether the incidence in neonatal jaundice had increased in the past 5 or 10 years and what the incidence of significant jaundice was in the unit in which the paediatrician worked.

Table 13.2　International survey on neonatal jaundice

Questionnaires mailed		Europe		North America	
		66		135	
Interim response		34 (51%)		63 (46%)	
Actively practising		26		40	
		a	b	a	b
1. Is the number of neonates who	Yes	5	4	5	6
develop significant jaundice* greater	No	8	15	15	21
now than in: (a) 1965, (b) 1970?	Uncertain	13	7	20	13
2. What do you estimate is the per-	Mean	15·8		12·2	
centage of neonates having	Range	2–30		3–30	
significant jaundice in 1975?					

* Significant jaundice was defined as a plasma bilirubin concentration ⩾ 12 mg/100 ml in the first 7 days after birth

In Europe 66 questionnaires were mailed to members of the European Society for Paediatric Research and in the USA 135 members of The

American Pediatric Society were included in the survey. Table 13.2 summarizes the interim results. Replies were analysed only from those respondents who stated that they were engaged in active practice in neonatal paediatrics. Of particular interest is that the majority of respondents in both Europe and USA stated that there had been no recent increase in the incidence of neonatal jaundice. It is also of interest that the estimated frequency of neonatal jaundice in different centres varies so widely, between 2 and 30% of neonates being estimated to develop significant jaundice, that is a serum bilirubin over 12 mg/100 ml. Nevertheless the mean estimate, 15·8% in Europe and 12·2% in the USA are very close to the published figures given in Table 13.1 for the percentage incidence of significant jaundice.

MATERNAL DRUGS AND JAUNDICE

There is little doubt that the use of drug therapy in obstetrics is increasing and it is natural that an association between maternal therapy and neonatal jaundice should be sought. In part, this association depends on whether a real increase in jaundice has occurred or not. As can be seen from the previous section this remains·an open question. It is certainly theoretically possible for maternal treatment before delivery to affect the serum bilirubin of the newborn infant. The possibility of treating neonates prenatally to reduce hyperbilirubinaemia has already been discussed in this volume (see Davies' chapter) and has been advocated as a routine therapy (Thomas, 1976). Another possibility is whether maternal drug therapy predisposes the infant in some way to neonatal jaundice.

The association of drugs and neonatal jaundice

The first specific association between maternal therapy and jaundice was made by Ghosh and Hudson (1972) who reported the incidence of jaundice in 197 neonates weighing over 5 lb born consecutively in 1972. In this group 6% of spontaneous delivered infants became jaundiced (< 12 mg/100 ml) while 9% of babies whose birth had been accelerated with oxytocin were jaundiced and 24% of those whose labours were induced with oxytocin became jaundiced.

Davies et al. (1973) studied 78 neonates prospectively. These were all healthy full-term babies and serum bilirubin was measured in each case on the 2nd and 5th day after birth. The mean concentration of bilirubin was higher on both occasions, 6·8 and 7·0 mg/100 ml respectively in the infants whose labours had been induced with oxytocin ($n = 36$) than in the spontaneous group ($n = 28$) 4·8 and 4·3 mg/100 ml respectively. The groups were similar in most other respects except that epidural anaesthesia was used in 66% of the induced group and 14% of the control group.

Chalmers et al. (1975) used data from 10 591 births registered on the Cardiff Birth Survey. Of 3326 infants born after oxytocin administration,

12·4% became jaundiced with a serum bilirubin greater than 10 mg/100 ml. Of 7265 infants born after spontaneous labour only 7·7% became jaundiced. At every gestational age apart from 36 weeks there was an increased incidence of jaundice in those infants born after oxytocin administration.

Beazley and Alderman (1975) studied 1353 neonates in a prospective study, measuring bilirubin at 3 and 6 days. They selected babies of 37 weeks gestation or more, weighing 2·5 kg or more at birth and delivered vaginally. Among those babies born after labour induced with oxytocin the incidence of jaundice was related to the dose of oxytocin used in the induction. The evidence of this relationship between oxytocin dose and jaundice is undermined however by the curiously high incidence of jaundice seen in those infants whose spontaneous labours were accelerated with oxytocin. The incidence of serum bilirubins over 12 mg/100 ml in the accelerated group was 16·1%, exceeding the incidence in the spontaneous no oxytocin group which was 6·3%, but also exceeding the incidence in the oxytocin induced group which was only 8·3%.

Campbell et al. (1975) compared the characteristics of 312 infants born in 1972 with unexplained peak bilirubin levels between 12 and 14 mg/100 ml with those of 312 matched infants who had not been jaundiced. The frequency of oxytocin administration to the mother was similar in both groups, but more of the mothers of the jaundiced children had had an epidural anaesthetic compared with the control, 55% compared with 45%. A weakness of this particular study is that the control and jaundiced groups were not matched for gestational age, 73% of the jaundiced group being under 40 weeks gestation as compared with 57% of the control group.

Sims and Neligan (1975) analysed 1032 births retrospectively and compared 46 jaundiced babies with bilirubins over 15 mg/100 ml with 92 control infants matched for sex and gestational age. More of the jaundiced infants had had labour induced with oxytocin, 52% versus 28%, and more had been born after an epidural anaesthetic, 39% versus 13%.

Friedman and Sachtleben (1976) reviewed 13 166 infants and found the incidence of jaundice, 10 mg/100 ml, correlated not with ocytocin use but with mid-forceps and breech extraction. This suggested that trauma was an important factor in the development of jaundice. It is possible that instrumental delivery may cause focal haemorrhages not readily detectable in the infant which lead to an increased bilirubin load to the neonatal liver.

Chew and Swann (1977) made a prospective study of 181 singleton deliveries. Bilirubins were measured on days 3 and 6. The mean serum bilirubin concentration was significantly higher in those babies whose deliveries were induced with oxytocin than in the group of babies born after spontaneous labour. Babies whose labour was accelerated but not induced with oxytocin had a mean serum bilirubin concentration no different to that in the spontaneous group. They found no relationship between the dose of oxytocin used and the serum bilirubin.

These results are very similar to those of Davies *et al.* (1973). Acceleration of labour was not associated with an increase in mean bilirubin levels on the 2nd and 5th day after birth, whereas induction of labour with oxytocin was so associated.

There is evidently a relationship between oxytocin use and neonatal jaundice although some workers have been unable to demonstrate it. The discrepancies may, in part, be methodological. It seems entirely reasonable to place more reliance on data obtained in prospective studies in which every child has had an estimation of serum bilirubin. This eliminates an important source of error, the failure to recognize raised bilirubin in a mildly jaundiced infant. Furthermore if oxytocin were affecting bilirubin metabolism, babies so exposed should show a shift in the mean bilirubin level rather than show a sporadic increase in the incidence of severe jaundice.

Three studies fulfil the criteria of prospective investigations with measurement of serum bilirubin in all infants (Beazley and Alderman, 1975; Chew and Swann, 1977; Davies *et al.*, 1973). These studies all suggest that induction of labour with oxytocin is icterogenic, and the mean increase in serum bilirubin is between 2 and 3 mg/100 ml.

Association of oxytocin, epidural anaesthetic and jaundice

In our retrospective survey of 12 543 singleton deliveries at Queen Charlotte's Hospital born between 1971 and 1976, we studied the association month by month between the incidence of serum bilirubins greater than 12 mg/100 ml and the oxytocin induction rate. This association is shown in Figure 13.2. There is a significant relationship, $P < 0.01$, between the induction rate and

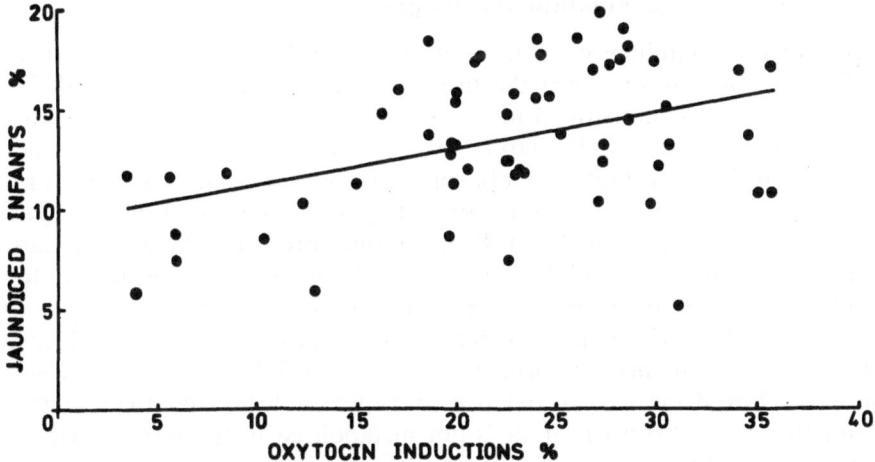

Figure 13.2 Relationship between oxytocin induction rate and jaundice rate (bilirubin > 11.9 mg/100 ml) between 1971 and 1975. Each point represents 1 month. $P < 0.01$

147

the incidence of jaundice. Similarly there was a significant correlation between the incidence of jaundice and the percentage of women receiving epidural anaesthetic. This association is shown in Figure 13.3. The correlation between epidural anaesthesia and jaundice is better than with oxytocin induction and jaundice.

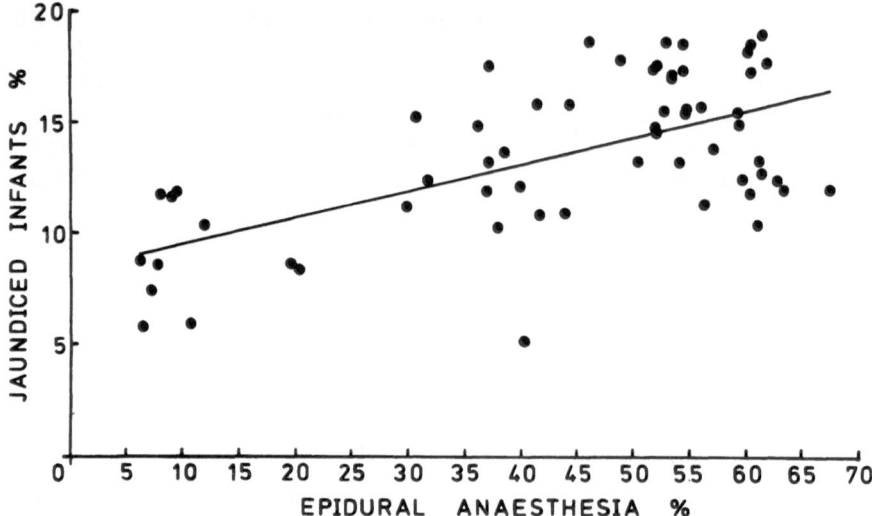

Figure 13.3 Relationship between epidural anaesthetic rate and jaundice rate (bilirubin > 11·9 mg/100 ml) between 1971 and 1975. Each point represents 1 month. $P < 0.01$

The effect of drugs on bilirubin conjugation

Many drugs can influence the metabolism of bilirubin. Inducing agents may accelerate the rate at which the liver can glucuronate bilirubin and this effect has been demonstrated in neonates for phenobarbitone given transplacentally (Thomas, 1976; Trolle, 1968). Other drugs may inhibit glucuronidation. The antibiotic novobiocin is a potent inhibitor of glucuronidation and for this reason is absolutely contraindicated in neonates (Hargreaves and Holton, 1962). Progesterones present in breast milk also inhibit the conjugation of bilirubin and are thought to be responsible for the slightly increased incidence of jaundice in breast fed infants.

It is thus theoretically possible for drugs given to the mother to influence the capacity of the neonatal liver to conjugate the bilirubin. It is not clear, however, how drugs such as oxytocin and epidural local anaesthetics might exert this effect. Oxytocin itself is not metabolized in the liver. However, bupivacaine, the amide local anaesthetic used most frequently in epidural anaesthesia, is metabolized in the liver and certain of its metabolites are glucuronated. Transfer of bupivacaine to the fetus does occur and it is possible that bupivacaine or its metabolites might compete for fetal glucu-ronyl transferase and thus competitively inhibit metabolism of bilirubin in the neonate.

The capacity of oxytocin and bupivacaine to inhibit glucuronidation was tested *in vitro* in the following manner. A suspension of microsomes was prepared from rat liver by differential centrifugation. The microsomal suspension prepared was equivalent to 0·5 g of liver per ml of incubate. The bilirubin UDP glucuronyl transferase activity of this preparation was measured using the method of Black and his co-workers (1970). The microsomal suspension was incubated with bilirubin and UDPGA at con-centrations of 64 μM and 7·29 mM respectively. To certain incubates, oxytocin, bupivacaine or novobiocin were added. Incubation was carried out at 37 °C for 30 min and the amount of bilirubin glucuronated by the liver preparation was measured by diazotization. In control experiments, the apparent K_m for UGDPA was 2·51 mM and for bilirubin it was 0·147 mM.

Table 13.3   Effect of drugs on bilirubin metabolism *in vitro*

Drug	Drug concentration	Bilirubin glucuronidation rate*
Control	—	59·2
Novobiocin	0·01 mM	18·0
Novobiocin	1·0 mM	3·4
Bupivacaine	0·01 mM	55·2
Bupivacaine	1·0 mM	54·1
Oxytocin	0·015 U/ml	59·7
Oxytocin	1·5 U/ml	59·7

* Rate is expressed as nmoles bilirubin conjugated per g liver per h

The effects of the drugs on this system are summarized in Table 13.3. It can be seen that novobiocin, a known inhibitor of glucuronyl transferase (Hargreaves and Holton, 1962), markedly decreased bilirubin conjugation. However neither bupivacaine nor oxytocin had any effect on the capacity of the liver microsomes to conjugate bilirubin. It is therefore unlikely that either of these drugs can exert a direct effect on bilirubin conjugation, but the possibility remains that metabolites of bupivacaine might exert a competitive effect.

SUMMARY

There are indications, although no definite proof, that neonates born in units practising active management of labour have an increased tendency to jaundice. The icterogenic effect of modern obstetrics is associated particu-larly with oxytocin induction of labour. However, it seems unlikely that oxytocin affects bilirubin metabolism in the neonate directly. Oxytocin does not interfere with glucuronidation of bilirubin *in vitro* and babies exposed to oxytocin during the course of spontaneous labour seem unaffected.

The most likely explanation of the icterogenic effect is that babies born after oxytocin induced labours are biochemically immature. Spontaneous labour is probably initiated by hormonal changes within the fetus rather than the mother. The child born after an induced labour has not undergone these hormonal changes and it is likely that metabolic consequences arise from this, one of which may be hepatic immaturity. The observation that the most severely jaundiced infants are those whose mothers received the largest doses of oxytocin supports this concept since the less responsive uterus is likely to contain the fetus whose hormonal response is least mature. The interposition of other factors known to influence hepatic maturation and bilirubin load such as early feeding, bruising, gestational age, breast feeding makes analysis of what is probably a minor influence difficult to confirm. The increasing use of prostaglandin induction of labour will probably enable a distinction to be made between the effect of the induction agent and the effect of the induction itself. It seems likely that it will be the induction *per se* which will be found ultimately responsible for the phenomenon of increased neonatal jaundice.

References

Beazley, J. M. and Alderman, B. (1975). Neonatal hyperbilirubinaemia following the use of oxytocin in labour. *Br. J. Obstet. Gynaecol.*, **82**, 265

Billing, B. H., Cole, P. G. and Lathe, G. H. (1954). Increased plasma bilirubin in newborn infants in relation to birthweight. *Br. Med. J.*, **2**, 1263

Black, M., Billing, B. H. and Heirwegh, K. P. M. (1970). Determination of bilirubin UDP glucuronyl transferase activity in needle biopsy specimens of human liver. *Clin. Chim. Acta*, **29**, 27

British Births 1970. (1975). Volume 1. (London: Heinemann)

Campbell, N., Harvey, D. and Norman, A. P. (1975). Increased frequency of neonatal jaundice in a maternity hospital. *Br. Med. J.*, **2**, 548

Chalmers, I., Campbell, H. and Turnbull, A. C. (1975). Use of oxytocin and incidence of neonatal jaundice. *Br. Med. J.*, **2**, 116

Chew, W. C. and Swann, I. L. (1977). Influence of simultaneous low amniotomy and oxytocin infusion and other maternal factors on neonatal jaundice: a prospective study. *Br. Med. J.*, **1**, 72

Dahms, B. B., Krauss, A. N., Gartner, L. M., Klain, D. B., Soodalter, J. and Auld, P. A. M. (1973). Breast feeding and serum bilirubin values during the first 4 days of life. *J. Paediatr.*, **83**, No. 6, 1049

Davidson, L. T., Merritt, K. K. and Weech, A. A. (1941). Hyperbilirubinemia in the newborn. *Am. J. Dis. Child.*, **61**, 958

Davies, D. P., Gomersall, R., Robertson, R., Gray, O. P. and Turnbull, A. C. (1973). Neonatal jaundice and maternal oxytocin infusion. *Br. Med. J.*, **3**, 476

Friedman, E. A. and Sachtleben, M. R. (1976). Neonatal jaundice in association with oxytocin stimulation of labour and operative delivery. *Br. Med. J.*, **1**, 198

Ghosh, A. and Hudson, F. P. (1972). Oxytocic agents and neonatal hyperbilirubinaemia. *Lancet*, **ii**, 823

Hargreaves, T. and Holton, J. B. (1962). Jaundice of the newborn due to novobiocin. *Lancet*, **i**, 839

Sims, D. G. and Neligan, G. A. (1975). Factors affecting the increasing incidence of severe non-haemolytic neonatal jaundice. *Br. J. Obstet. Gynaecol.*, **82**, 863

Thomas, C. R. (1976). Routine phenobarbital for prevention of neonatal hyperbilirubinemia. *Obstet. Gynecol.*, **47**, No. 3, 304

Trolle, D. (1968). Decrease of total serum bilirubin concentration in newborn infants after phenobarbitone treatment. *Lancet*, **ii**, 705

Zuelzer, W. W. and Brown, A. K. (1961). Neonatal jaundice. *Am. J. Dis. Child.*, **101**, 87

14
The Influence of Maternal Drug Administration on Human Fetal Breathing Movements *in utero*

K. BODDY

Previous experiments in sheep have shown that the irregular episodic breathing movements of the fetus *in utero*, are more susceptible to pentobarbitone than the more regular maintained breathing seen after birth (Boddy *et al.*, 1976). In these studies complex age and time related responses were seen in the fetal electrocortical and breathing activities as well as in the fetal circulation. The dose of pentobarbitone administered intravenously to the ewe (4 mg/kg), was only sufficient to cause light maternal sedation. It cannot therefore be assumed that drugs used for maternal sedation in human pregnancy are without significant consequences for the fetus.

Drugs influencing the autonomic nervous system have also been shown to produce quantitatively different responses in the fetus compared to the adult (van Petten, 1975). Such considerations may be important when choosing drugs for control of maternal hypertension, and it is clear that more precise information of their effects on the fetus is required.

In human pregnancy, fetal chest-wall movements have been recorded using A-scan ultrasound (Boddy and Robinson, 1971). Maternal administration of pethidine (100 mg i.m.) and diazepam (10 mg i.v.) has been seen to result in an arrest of fetal breathing activity. In mothers receiving long-term repeated doses of barbiturates, diazepam or the anticonvulsant phenytoin sodium (Epanutin), recordings have been obtained of fetal breathing movements which were normal in incidence and character (Boddy, 1976). Such recordings did not take into account time-related responses and measurements of drug concentrations were not made. Subsequent studies have now

Table 14.1 The effect of maternal administration of respiratory depressant drugs on normal fetal breathing movements *in utero* (mild hyptertension in pregnancy)

	Drug	Initial dose (mg)	Maternal sedation	Weeks gestation	No.	% Incidence of fetal breathing movements				Subsequent oral dose (mg Qds)
						Prior	Immediate response	2nd hour	Day 1–3	
Oral	Na amytal	200	mild	≤ 30 weeks	3	40 ± 10	variable	10 ± 10	35 ± 10	200
				≥ 32 weeks	5	60 ± 10	variable	40 ± 10	55 ± 10	200
	sparine	100	mild	≥ 32 weeks	5	70 ± 10	variable	40 ± 10	60 ± 10	100
	diazepam	20	mild	≥ 32 weeks	5	65 ± 10	variable	20 ± 10	60 ± 10	10
i.m.	Na amytal	200	mild-moderate	≥ 32 weeks	5	65 ± 10	variable	40 ± 10	60 ± 10	200
	sparine	100	moderate	≥ 32 weeks	5	60 ± 10	variable	35 ± 10	65 ± 10	100
	diazepam	20	moderate	≤ 30 weeks	2	< 35 / 30	apnoea (15–60 min)	< 10 / 10	< 10 / 10	10
				≥ 32 weeks	5	60 ± 10	variable	30 ± 10	55 ± 10	10

been made to investigate the influence and time-related responses of maternal drug administration on fetal breathing movements in human pregnancy. Two types of drugs have been used, namely the respiratory depressants (sodium amytal; sparine; diazepam and pethidine), and the anti-hypertensive methyldopa. Only patients requiring these drugs in the management of their pregnancies have been studied. In all but three patients, however, the incidence and character of the fetal breathing movements were normal before drug administration. Recordings were made using A-scan ultrasound, 1½ hours before and for 2 hours after drug administration. Subsequently recordings of 1½ hours duration were made on each of the three successive days following the initial dose of drug.

A variety of influences are known to affect fetal breathing movements *in utero*, e.g. maternal smoking, overnight starvation, exercise and abdominal palpation. Also changes occur with increasing gestation and with time of day (Boddy *et al.*, 1973; Boddy, 1976). Adverse factors were avoided in the present work and recordings were only made between 9.00 a.m. and 1.30 p.m.

Table 14.1 shows the effect of maternally administered respiratory depressant drugs on previously normal fetal breathing activity. The gestational ages of these pregnancies ranged from 28 weeks to 42 weeks (mean 36 weeks) from the last normal menstrual period. All were complicated by mild hypertension without proteinuria (mean systolic blood-pressure 145 ± 5 mmHg; mean diastolic blood-pressure 90 ± 5 mmHg). A reduced mean incidence of breathing movements was seen in the second hour after drug administration in all fetuses. All patients continued to receive an oral dose of the respiratory depressant drug but the incidence of fetal breathing activity on each of the three days succeeding was not significantly different from that prior to the initial dose. This was so except in the two patients receiving diazepam with pregnancies less than 31 weeks gestation. The reduced mean incidence of fetal breathing seen following oral administration of sodium amytal, was not considered significant, except in three instances where the gestational ages were also below 31 weeks. These results suggest that the drugs studied crossed the placenta in sufficient amounts to influence the fetal central nervous system and reduce the incidence of breathing movements even though only mild to moderate sedation was achieved in the mother. They are in accord with previous results in sheep and indicate the vulnerability of the fetus before the 32nd week of pregnancy and to diazepam compared with sodium amytal or sparine. There were no significant differences between oral or intra-muscular administration of these drugs. In five pregnancies complicated by hypertension and significant proteinuria, administration of 10 mg of diazepam by the i.v. route had a profound effect on the incidence of fetal breathing movements (Figure 14.1). Intramuscular pethidine (100 mg) given to five patients prior to removal of a cervical suture, was also followed by an initial decrease in fetal breathing activity, but the mean incidence of fetal breathing movements in those patients receiving oral sodium amytal, sparine or diazepam after the 33rd week of pregnancy was only reduced in the latter half of the 2nd hour after drug administration. In all instances, however, the initial effect was relatively short lived except in the five pregnancies receiving diazepam (Figure 14.1). The placental transfer of diazepam has been demonstrated in human pregnancy and higher drug concentrations have been found in umbilical cord plasma than in maternal plasma after equilibrium had been obtained (Cavanagh and Condo, 1964; Shannon *et al.*, 1972; Cree *et al.*, 1973). The drug is cleared slowly from the fetal brain in contrast to other tissues and does not rapidly equilibrate with other fetal compartments once localized in the central nervous system.

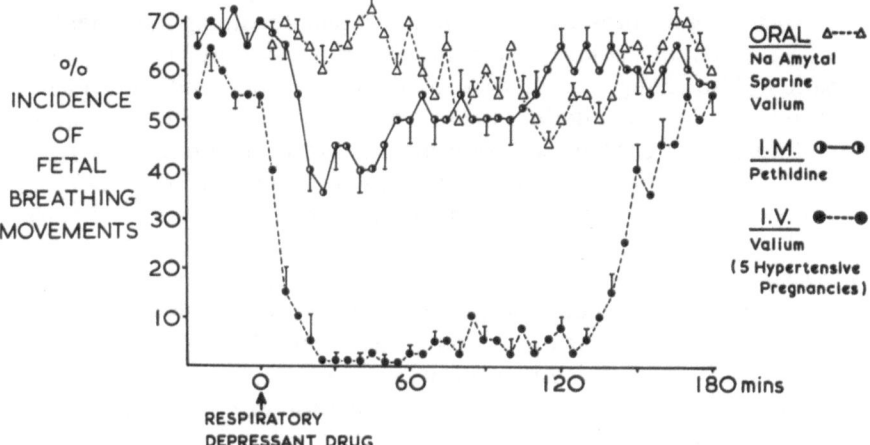

Figure 14.1 Maternal administration of respiratory depressant drugs: 34–42 weeks' gestation —normal breathing activity

Moreover, the human fetus is unable to metabolize diazepam to any appreciable extent, and even after delivery the parent compound and its active metabolites may not be cleared for up to 1 week (Cree *et al.*, 1973). It is not surprising therefore that the effects of maternal administration of diazepam on human fetal breathing activity *in utero* were more marked and more prolonged than those of the other drugs studied and particularly so in the younger fetuses. The smaller effect and quicker recovery seen following i.m. administration of diazepam may be accounted for by the poorer absorption and lower maternal blood levels achieved by this route. It is interesting to speculate on the reasons which may account for a normal incidence of fetal breathing activity in pregnancies where regular repeated ingestion of diazepam has occurred over several weeks, and for the return of normal amounts of breathing movements seen in more mature fetuses in the present studies. Despite the inability of the human fetus to *N*-demethylate and conjugate diazepam, adaptation may occur as it does in adults subjected to repeated administration of respiratory depressant drugs. It is also possible that enzyme induction may occur with repeated dosage and the inability of the immature liver to respond within the period of observation may account for the differences observed between the younger and older fetuses (see Chapter 12). It is evident from these preliminary results that respiratory depressant drugs administered to mothers during pregnancy require extended study to determine their short- and long-term effects on the fetus. The ability to record fetal breathing movements *in utero* provides a useful tool for such studies.

The pharmacological action and effects of methyldopa (aldomet) in human pregnancy are little understood. The placental transfer of several different β-receptor blocking agents has been documented in animal studies (Truelove *et al.*, 1973; van Petten and Willes, 1970; van Petten and McCracken, 1973; van Petten, 1975). In the presence of B-blockade the ability of the fetus to respond to adverse conditions such as asphyxia will be severely impaired. The recent evidence that propranolol may produce full β-blockade in the fetus, of three times longer duration than that seen in the mother, and reports of bradycardia in neonates whose mothers received propranolol for thyrotoxicosis during pregnancy, suggest cause for concern. In the present studies human fetal breathing movements were recorded in eight pregnancies complicated by essential hypertension. Aldomet was used to control the hypertension, the initial dose being given between 30 and 32 weeks' gestation. In three patients the incidence of fetal breathing movements was reduced before starting treatment with aldomet. Figure 14.2 shows the mean incidence

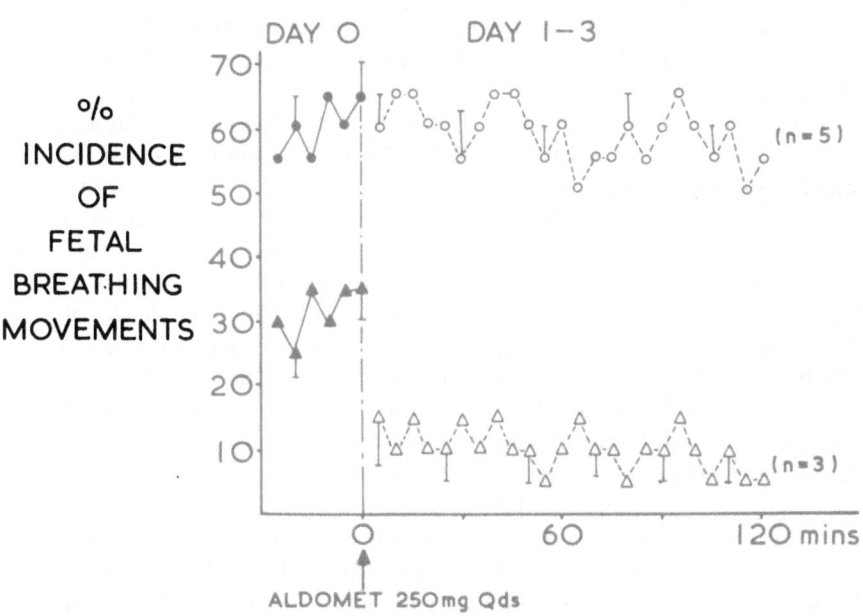

Figure 14.2 Effect of methyldopa on fetal breathing movements *in utero*: eight hypertensive pregnancies—30–32 weeks' gestation

of breathing movements before treatment and on the first 3 days after the initial dose of aldomet. No change in the mean incidence was seen in the five pregnancies where the amount of fetal breathing activity was considered to be normal before treatment. A significant further reduction of this activity was observed however in the other three fetuses. Table 14.2 shows that there were no significant differences between these two groups of patients

Table 14.2   Effect of aldomet on normal fetal breathing movements

					Incidence of fetal breathing movement				
No.	Mean B.P. prior to aldomet (4 readings)		Mean B.P. day 1–3 (18 readings)		Prior to aldomet	Day 1–3	SB	NND	Fetal distress in labour
	Systolic	Diastolic	Systolic	Diastolic					
5	155	100	135	85	60%	55%	0	0	0 (1 LSCS)
3	155	100	140	80	35%	10%	1 (APH)	0	2 (LSCS)

in their initial blood-pressure recordings or the reduction achieved by treatment. In all instances the dose and route of administration of aldomet was the same (250 mg/t.d.s. by the oral route). One of the three pregnancies in which the incidence of fetal breathing movements was reduced, was significantly different in that urinary protein was present, from the 34th week (never more than 2 g/24 hours).

This pregnancy subsequently terminated at the 36th week with a sudden accidental haemorrhage and still-birth. All the remaining patients had no more than an occasional trace of urinary protein and were allowed to labour (gestational ages 37–39 weeks). Their babies were all live born, above the 10th centile weight for gestation and there were no first-week deaths. Fetal distress in labour, requiring lower segment Caesarean section, occurred in three instances. Only one of these showed a normal incidence of fetal breathing movements following treatment with aldomet (Table 14.2). The small number of patients so far studied allows no firm conclusions to be made. A reduced amount of fetal breathing movements, recorded with due regard to the multifactorial control of these movements, has previously been associated with a deteriorating fetal condition and an increased incidence of fetal distress in labour (Boddy, 1976). The cause for the reduced incidence seen following administration of aldomet is most likely due to effects of this drug on the fetal circulation and/or the placental circulation. This would be in accord with what is known concerning the effects of adrenoceptor antagonists such as propranolol (van Petten, 1975; Tunstall, 1969). It is unlikely that a central action of aldomet directly influencing fetal breathing movements would account for the present observations. If these conclusions are allowed then it is essential that more precise and additional information is required before such potentially dangerous drugs become widely used in obstetric practice.

References

Boddy, K. (1976). In R. W. Beard and P. W. Nathanielsz (eds.). *Fetal Circulation and Breathing Movements, Fetal Physiology and Medicine*, pp. 302–328. (London, Philadelphia and Toronto: W. B. Saunders)

Boddy, K. and Robinson, J. S. (1971). External method for detection of fetal breathing *in utero*. *Lancet*, **ii**, 1231

Boddy, K., Dawes, G. S. and Robinson, J. S. (1973). A 24-hour rhythm in the fetus. In R. S. Comline, K. W. Cross, G. S. Dawes and P. W. Nathanielsz (eds.) *Foetal and Neonatal Physiology*, pp. 63–66. (London: Cambridge University Press)

Boddy, K., Dawes, G. S., Fischer, R. L., Pinter, S. and Robinson, J. S. (1976). The effects of pentobarbitone and pethidine on fetal breathing movements in sheep. *J. Physiol.*

Cavanagh, D. and Condo, C. S. (1964). *Curr. Ther. Res.*, **6**, 122

Cree, J. E., Meyer, J. and Hailey, D. M. (1973). Diazepam in labour: its metabolism and effect on the clinical condition and thermogenesis of the newborn. *Br. Med. J.*, **4**, 251

Shannon, R. W., Fraser, G. P., Aitken, R. G. and Harper, J. R. (1972). *Br. J. Clin. Pract.*, **26**, 271

Truelove, J. F., van Petten, G. R. and Willes, R. F. (1973). *Br. J. Pharmacol.*, **47**, 161

Tunstall, M. E. (1969). The effect of propranolol on the onset of breathing at birth. *Br. J. Anaesth.*, **41**, 792

van Petten, G. R. (1975). Pharmacology and the fetus. *Br. Med. Bull.*, **31**, 75

van Petten, G. R. and McCracken. (1973). *Clin. Res.*, **20**, 914 (abstract)

van Petten, G. R. and Willes, R. F. (1970). β-adrenoceptive responses in the unanaesthetized ovine fetus. *Br. J. Pharmacol.*, **38**, 572

Discussion

Mucklow: It was suggested to us earlier on that diazepam given intravenously is the drug of choice in the treatment of status epilepticus in pregnancy as indeed it is in non-pregnant individuals. In view of the fact you've shown it depresses fetal breathing activity and hence probably fetal central nervous system activity would you like to comment on this?

Boddy: When I first saw the response to diazepam given intravenously I was worried. But when I examined these fetuses again several days later they all seem to be coming back into the normal range. I am reassured by the fetus accommodating to the effect so readily. Immediate delivery following intravenous maternal administration of diazepam may however have serious consequences.

Herxheimer: Do you ever give diazepam twice to one mother so that you can see whether you get this effect on second occasions?

Boddy: Yes we have done this and in fact you do not get as great a response on the second occasion.

Beilin: I would like to ask how many of the cases you presented treated with methyldopa were ones that you studied in Oxford?

Boddy: None of them were the ones I studied in Oxford.

Lewis: What happened to the women in Oxford, Dr Beilin?

Beilin: The point of my question was really to ask what other signs of hypertension these women had when they were treated with methyldopa. I remember that several of the women studied with methyldopa at Oxford were deteriorating in their general clinical condition at the time the methyldopa was started, this raises the problem of how much of the deterioration of fetal breathing was due to the methyldopa and how much was due to their underlying condition.

Boddy: In the cases I presented there was no deterioration in maternal condition that required any active management. Most of them went on to 37–38 weeks gestation and the study I showed was carried out between 28 and 32 weeks. We followed all these pregnancies through from the 32nd to the 38th week. We noted that the fetal breathing activity remained low during that time, but there were no clinical indications for interference.

Dawes: What method are you using? The A-scan method?

Boddy: Yes, all these observations were made using the A-scan.

Dawes: Do you have any similar results using real time scanning?

Boddy: We didn't use real time scanning but we have used the pulsed-doppler method in parallel with A-scan and recorded identical incidences of fetal breathing movements (In press). There are problems with real-time scanning in that small amplitude movements are not readily visualized due to poor resolution, and the large multiple array transducers are unsuitable for long-term continuous recording.

Boddy: I wonder if I could ask you, Professor Dawes, what do you think of the idea that the methyldopa is having an effect on the fetal circulation and that the reduction in fetal breathing is secondary to this. I recall when we did our experiments with pentobarbitone we did not think that the circulatory effects of the drug on the fetus were sufficient to explain the effect on the fetal respiratory movements.

Dawes: In the pentobarbitone experiments in the sheep, pentobarbitone did not alter the blood gases of the fetus. It was therefore very unlikely that the hypoxia was responsible for the effect on fetal breathing. However, in the human we do not know what methyldopa does, indeed we do not know what methyldopa does in the fetal sheep.

Boddy: I can say that the blood gases of these babies were all normal at delivery.

Dawes: There is in fact no evidence that methyldopa adversely effects the fetus but I am just saying that nobody has actually made the critical observations.

Index

Abortion 56–7, 58
  infection after 73
  methyldopa administration 158
Aldomet, *see* Methyldopa
Alpha-adrenoceptor blockers 39–40
Alpha-methyldopa 9–10
Amiloride hydrochloride 48
Aminopterin 113
Ampicillin 76, 77
Amylobarbitone 129, 132
Anaesthesia, epidural 30, 146, 147–8
Anoxia 50
Antibiotic prophylaxis 75–7, 80
Anticoagulant therapy 82 ff
Anticonvulsant therapy (epilepsy) 105,
  106–8, 109 ff
Antipyrine 129, 130, 131–2
Arterial changes (hypertension) 20, 21
Asphyxia, fetal 60
Atenolol 37, 38
Autonomic nervous system 39, 41

Bacteraemia 72, 73
  streptococcal, *see* Streptococcal transient
Bacterial endocarditis 70, 80
Bacteriuria, asymptomatic 12–13
Barbiturates 26, 44, 57, 113
  see also Barbiturates by name
Bed rest (hypertension) 2, 4, 25–6, 56
Benzo-(a)-pyrene hydroxylase 129, 130, 131,
  133
Benzodiazepine 107
Beta-adrenergic blockade 14, 45, 50, 157
Beta-adrenoceptor antagonists 36–7
Beta-blockers 37–9, 41, 42, 61, 65
Betamethasone 42
Beta-sympathomimetics 29–30
Bethanidine 11, 48, 58, 59, 60
Bilirubin 130, 138–9, 141
  jaundice 141 ff
Birthweight 5–6
  hyperthyroidism 97
  jaundice 143
Bleeding
  anticoagulant therapy 83–6
  anticonvulsant therapy 114
Bradycardia 14, 37, 157
Breast feeding
  anticonvulsant therapy 107
  carbimazole therapy 96

  progesterones (jaundice) 148
  warfarin therapy 87
British Births Survey (1970) (jaundice) 143–4
Bupivacaine 148–9

Caesarian section 31
  bleeding 84
  diabetes mellitus 121
  methyldopa administration 8, 9, 158
Carbamazepine 106
Carbimazole 95, 96, 97, 98
Cardiac surgery 69–70
Catecholamines 36–7, 38, 64
Catheter fever 73
Cephaloridine 76
Cephalexin 76
Chlorpromazine (CPZ) 31, 131, 132
Chlorthiazide 28
Cigarette smoking 131
Circulation, placental (hypertension) 22 ff,
  28, 39–42
Cleft lip and palate 109, 112, 113
Clonazepam 107
Clonidine 11, 30, 48, 58, 59, 60
Colloid goitre 99
Congenital heart disease 69 ff, 98
  epilepsy 109, 113
  incidence 69–70
Congenital malformations
  diabetes mellitus 118, 122–3
  epilepsy 109 ff
Contraceptive pill 82
Cord thyroid hormone levels 94, 95, 97
Crystalline penicillin 76
Cyanide injections 39
Cystic nodular goitre 99
Cytochrome P-450 127–8, 130, 134, 135

Death, perinatal
  diabetes mellitus 117, 122
  endocarditis 71
  hypertension 53–4
  propranolol treatment 47, 48, 49, 52
  thyrotoxicosis, neonatal 98
Debrisoquine 11, 48, 59, 60
N-Demethylase 129, 131, 156
Dexamethasone 42, 121
Diazepam 26, 57
  breathing, fetal 153–6. 160
  epilepsy 107–8

163

Diazoxide 14, 28
Diuretics 11, 14, 28, 57–8, 59, 60, 61
  see also Thiazide
Drug metabolism 127–9, 134–5
  respiratory depressant drugs 156–7

Eclampsia 107
Endocarditis 70 ff
Enterococcal endocarditis 74
Enzymes
  drug metabolizing 127, 128–30, 138
  hydroxylating (anticonvulsant drugs) 106
Epidural anaesthetic (jaundice) 146, 147–8
Epoxide hydrase (trichloropropene oxide)
  135
Erythromycin therapy (endocarditis) 76
Ethylmorphine 128, 129
Euthyroid state of pregnancy 94, 95, 96, 97,
  100
Extraction, tooth (endocarditis) 72–3

Fetotoxicities 134
Fick principle 23
'First pass' (drug metabolism) 134
Folate deficiency 113, 114
Folic acid deficiency (epilepsy) 113, 114
Free triiodothyronine index (FT_3I) 94, 97, 99
Free thyroxine index (FT_4I) 94–5, 96, 97, 98,
  99, 100
Frusemide 28

Ganglion blockers 26
Genetics (epilepsy) 103–4, 113, 115
Genital tract infection 73–4
Gentamycin 76, 77
Gilbert's syndrome 130
Glucose levels, blood (diabetes mellitus) 118,
  120, 122–3
Glucuronidation (jaundice) 148–9
Glucuronyl transferase 130
  jaundice 149
Glycosuria 119–20
Goitre, see Goitres by name
Graves' disease 97, 98
Guanethidine 11, 27, 48

Haemodynamics of hypertension 20–2
Haemorrhage, post-partum 83–6, 87
Hashimoto's thyroiditis 100
Heparin, subcutaneous 83, 84, 85–6, 89
Hexamethonium 25
Hexobarbitone 130–1
Hydrallazine 9, 10, 27, 31, 48, 49, 61, 108
Hydrochlorthiazide 48
Hydroxylating enzymes 106, 138
Hyperglycaemia 117–18
Hyperinsulinism 118
Hyperthyroidism 93, 95 ff, 98

neonatal 97–8
surgical treatment 96
Hypoglycaemia 37, 118, 120, 121, 122
Hypotensive drugs 24–5
Hypothyroidism 98–9, 102
Hypoxia, fetal 38–9, 50, 65

Immunoglobulins, thyroid stimulating 97–8
Indomethacin 42
Induced labour (jaundice) 150
Infective endocarditis 70–1
Infertility (hypothyroidism) 98
Insecticides 138
Insulin 118, 120–1
Iodized salt 99
Isophane insulin 120
Isoprenaline 29, 37
Isotope scanning, thyroid 99
Isoxuprine 30

Jaundice, incidence of 141–5

Kernicterus 141

Lactation (anticoagulant therapy) 85
Liver, fetal (enzyme induction) 133
Long-acting thyroid stimulator-projector
  (LATS-P) 97–8

Magnesium sulphate 108
Menorrhagia (hypothyroidism) 99
Methyldopa 3, 4, 5, 8–9, 15, 18, 25, 27–8, 31,
  45, 48, 57–8, 59, 60, 61, 63, 64, 65, 157–8,
  160, 161
N-Methylaniline 128, 130
Metoprolol 37, 38
Microcephaly (anticoagulant therapy) 86
Micro-organisms (endocarditis) 72–7
Milk, mother's, see Breast feeding
Mitral regurgitation 71
Mortality, see Death, perinatal
Multinodular goitre 95, 99
Myometrium 21
  drugs, response to 22, 23

NADPH-cytochrome c reductase,
  see Cytochrome P-450
Neonatal hyperthyroidism 97–8
Neurone blocking agents, sympathetic 11
P-Nitrobenzoic acid (PNA) 132
Nodular goitre 99–100
Non-eclamptic seizures during pregnancy
  104
Novobiocin 148, 149

Oedema 20
Optic atrophy (anticoagulant therapy) 86
Orciprenaline 29

Oxytocin administration (jaundice) 145–6, 147–50

5 (Parahydroxyphenyl)-5-phenylhydanton 106
Pathology (hypertension) 20
Penicillin therapy (endocarditis) 70–1, 76–7
Pentobarbitone 40–1, 44, 153, 161
Pentolinium 48
Periapical lesions 72
Peridontal disease (endocarditis) 72
Perineal tears 84, 89
Pethidine 153, 155
Pheneturide 106
Phenindione 87
Phenobarbitone 44, 107, 112, 130, 131, 133, 148
Phenytoin 106–7, 112–13, 129, 134–5, 153
Placental transfer
  anticonvulsant drugs 112
  enzyme induction 129–33
  respiratory depressant drugs 155–6
  thyroid hormones 94, 95
Post-partum haemorrhage 84–6, 87, 89
Post-partum infection 73–4, 75
Practolol 14, 37, 38
Pre-eclampsia 1, 2, 4, 8, 15, 19–20, 31, 48
  diuretics 12, 13
  hypotensive drugs 25
  propranolol treatment 47–8
Progesterones (jaundice) 148
Propranolol 14, 29, 36, 37, 38, 41, 45 ff, 157, 158–9
Propyl thiouracil 97
Prostaglandin induced labour (jaundice) 150
Prostaglandin synthetase inhibition 42
Proteinuria 1, 2, 3, 8, 19
  propranolol treatment 47, 48, 52
  respiratory depressant drugs 155
Protoveratine 26, 31
Pyorrhoea (endocarditis) 72

Radioactive testing (reaction to anti-hypertensive drugs) 23, 29
Rauwolfia alkaloids, see Reserpine
Reactive epoxide 134–5
Reserpine 11, 26–7, 48, 49, 59, 60
Rheumatic heart disease 69 ff, 98
  incidence 70
Ritodrine 29, 30
Root canals, infected tooth (endocarditis) 72

Salbutamol 14
Sedatives 14, 26
Seizures, epileptic, during pregnancy 104, 105
Sepsis, dental (endocarditis) 73
Side effects
  anticoagulant therapy 86

anticonvulsant therapy 106, 109
antihypertensive drugs 8–11, 13, 28
propranolol 49–50
respiratory depressant drugs 155
Skeletal abnormalities (epileptic mothers) 111, 112
Sodium amytal 154, 155, 156
Soluble insulin 120
Sotalol 37, 38
Sparine 154, 155, 156
Staphylococcal infection (endocarditis) 72, 73, 74
Status epilepticus 107, 108
Streptococcal bacteraemia, transient 72, 73, 74, 75–6
Streptococcus viridans 73, 74–5, 76, 77
Streptomycin 76, 77
Sulthiame 106

Teeth, infected (endocarditis) 71–3
Teratogenicity
  anticoagulant therapy (warfarin) 83, 86
  anticonvulsant therapy 111–13, 114, 134–5
  hypoglycaemic drugs, oral 121
Termination of pregnancy, see Abortion
2,3,7,8-Tetrachlorodibenzo-p-dioxin (TCDD) 133, 138
'Thermistor' needle probe 23–4, 29
Thermogenesis 36
Thiazide 4, 13, 45
Thromboembolism, risk of, in pregnancy 82
Thyroid binding globulin (TBG) 102
Thyroidectomy, partial 96, 97
Thyroid hormones 93 ff
Thyroid stimulating hormone (TSH) 94, 95, 97, 98, 102
Thyrotoxicosis, neonatal 97–8, 102
Thyrotophin 93
Thyroxine (T_4) 94, 95, 96, 99, 102
L-Thyroxine 96, 97, 98, 100
Thyroxine-binding globulin (TBG) 93–4, 95
Tonsillitis 73
Toxaemia 28, 58
Tranquilizing drugs 14
Triiodothyronine (T_3) 94, 99
Triiodothyronine resin uptake (T_3RU) 94

Ultrasound
  breathing movements, fetal 154, 155, 160
  diabetes mellitus 121
  thyroid 99

Vasoconstriction 39–40
Vasodilators, see Hydrallazine
Vitamin K therapy 114

Warfarin 83, 84–5